SOCIAL PSYCHOLOGY AND HEALTH

MAPPING SOCIAL PSYCHOLOGY SERIES
Series Editor: Tony Manstead

Current titles:

Icek Ajzen: Attitudes, Personality, and Behavior
Robert S. Baron, Norbert L. Kerr, and Norman Miller: Group Process,
   Group Decision, Group Action
Steve Duck: Relating to Others
J. Richard Eiser: Social Judgment
Russell G. Geen: Human Aggression
Howard Giles and Nikolas Coupland: Language: Contexts and
   Consequences
Dean G. Pruitt and Peter J. Carnevale: Negotiation in Social Conflict
Wolfgang Stroebe and Margaret S. Stroebe: Social Psychology and Health
John C. Turner: Social Influence
Leslie A. Zebrowitz: Social Perception

Forthcoming titles:

Marilynn B. Brewer and Norman Miller: Intergroup Relations
Miles Hewstone and Neil Macrae: Stereotyping and Social Cognition
Richard Petty: Attitude Change

SOCIAL PSYCHOLOGY AND HEALTH

Wolfgang Stroebe
Margaret S. Stroebe

Brooks/Cole Publishing Company

I(T)P™ An International Thomson Publishing Company

Pacific Grove • Albany • Bonn • Boston • Cincinnati • Detroit
London • Madrid • Melbourne • Mexico City • New York • Paris
San Francisco • Singapore • Tokyo • Toronto • Washington

Dedicated to our daughter
Katherine Stroebe

Open University Press
Celtic Court
22 Ballmoor
Buckingham MK18 1XW

First Published 1995

This U.S. edition published in 1995 by
Brooks/Cole Publishing Company
A Division of International Thomson Publishing Inc.
511 Forest Lodge Road
Pacific Grove, CA 93950

Library of Congress Cataloging-in-Publication Data

Stroebe, Wolfgang.
    Social psychology and health / Wolfgang Stroebe and Margaret S.
Stroebe.
        p. cm. — (Mapping social psychology series)
    Includes bibliographical references and index.
    ISBN 0-534-26004-7
    1. Clinical health psychology.   I. Stroebe, Margaret S.
II. Title.   III. Series.
R726.7.S78   1995   95-3089
155.9′16—dc20   CIP

Typeset by Graphicraft Typesetters Limited, Hong Kong
Printed and bound in the United States by Malloy Lithographing, Inc.
Ann Arbor, Michigan

CONTENTS

FOREWORD

There has long been a need for a carefully tailored series of reasonably short and inexpensive books on major topics in social psychology, written primarily for students by authors who enjoy a reputation for the excellence of their research and their ability to communicate clearly and comprehensibly their knowledge of, and enthusiasm for, the discipline. The *Mapping Social Psychology* series has been designed to meet that need. The aim of each volume in the series is to provide a concise and up-to-date overview of the concepts, theories, methods, and findings relating to a key topic in social psychology. Although the intention is to produce books that will be used by senior-level undergraduates and graduate students, the fact that the books are written in a straightforward style should also make them accessible to newcomers to social psychology. At the same time, the books are intended to be sufficiently informative and up-to-date to earn the respect of researchers and instructors.

The rationale for this series is twofold. First, conventional textbooks are too low-level and uninformative for use with senior undergraduates or graduate students. Books in this series *address* this problem partly by dealing with key topics at book length, rather than chapter length, and partly by the fact that each book is authored by an acknowledged expert on the topic in question. Second, traditional textbooks are often dependent on research conducted in or examples drawn from North American society. This fosters the mistaken impression that social psychology is an exclusively North American discipline, and can also be baffling for readers who are unfamiliar with North American culture. To combat this problem, authors of books in this series have been encouraged to adopt a broader perspective, citing examples and research from outside North America wherever this is appropriate. The aim is to produce a series for a world market, introducing readers to an international discipline.

Health has become a major topic in psychology during the past two decades. Much of this research and theorizing concerning health has been social psychological in nature, reflecting the growing awareness that health in modern industrialized societies is determined to a large degree by behaviors that are either voluntarily committed (for example, smoking) or voluntarily withheld (for example, physical exercise). Understanding the determinants of these health-related behaviors is a prime task for social psychologists. Equally, identifying the most effective means by which such behaviors may be modified has attracted a great deal of attention from social psychologists. Finally, there has also been an increasing awareness of the extent to which health is influenced by the social network within which one lives. Personal relationships provide us with important resources for coping with the ordinary and extraordinary stresses of everyday life. Here is another way in which social psychology contributes to the understanding of health and illness.

In this book Wolfgang and Margaret Stroebe provide us with a scholarly yet highly readable account of how social psychology contributes to the understanding and modification of health-related behaviors, and also of how these processes of understanding and modification sometimes force social psychologists to re-evaluate their favorite tenets. The authors focus on a number of key questions: What exactly are the health risks associated with certain kinds of behavior? Why do people engage in such health-impairing behaviors, and what can be done to reduce them? What are the benefits associated with self-protective behaviors, and what can be done to encourage them? What are the health consequences of psychosocial stress? What are the personal and social factors that moderate and mediate the relationship between stress and ill health? Throughout the book, the authors pay careful attention both to what is known about health, on the basis of epidemiological and clinical research, and to what is known about the determinants of the associated risk behaviors, on the basis of social psychological theory and research. Theoretical points are clearly developed and the link with what is known about health is carefully explained. Because the topic of health is so inherently interesting – but also because the way the book is written is so inviting – this is a book that readers of all kinds are likely to enjoy. It will be an outstanding resource for social psychologists who are interested in knowing more about how their discipline can address key issues in health and for health professionals who are interested in knowing more about the principles and methods of social psychology.

Tony Manstead
Series Editor

PREFACE

Much of health psychology is applied social psychology. So much so that a thorough discussion of all the areas in which social psychology has made contributions to health psychology would not have been possible within the page constraints of this series. Faced with the choice between attempting a complete but necessarily superficial review of the whole social psychology of health or an in-depth analysis of selected areas, we opted for the latter alternative. We decided to focus on two areas which are of major importance for both health psychology and social psychology, namely the areas of health behavior and psychosocial stress.

The study of health behavior is based on two assumptions: First, that at least in industrial societies, a substantial proportion of the mortality from the leading causes of death is due to health-impairing behavior patterns, and second, that these behavior patterns are modifiable. Evidence for the health-impairing nature of various behavior patterns is provided by epidemiological studies, an area of research which would normally not be considered relevant to social psychology. However, since it would make little sense to design mass media campaigns to change a given behavior unless it were proven to be unhealthy, part of our discussion of health behavior is devoted to an analysis of these epidemiological findings.

Evidence on the modifiability of health-impairing behavior patterns comes from the assessment of interventions aimed at changing health behavior. One first important step in developing such interventions, which in practice is often omitted, is the analysis of the psychological factors which determine this behavior. One lesson to be learned from this research is that the general custom to design campaigns on the basis of common sense may be one of the reasons why health education is often not very effective. For example, educational campaigns on sexual risk behavior still emphasize knowledge about the risk of HIV infection and the severity of contracting such infections. Studies of sexually active students, on the other hand, do not find that their intentions to use condoms are strongly influenced by these factors. Instead, students seem to be concerned about perceived barriers to condom use, such as beliefs concerning pleasure reduction or awkwardness of use.

But even if health education is effective in persuading people to change health impairing life styles, people often fail to act according to their intentions. Thus, the probability of smokers stopping smoking at their first attempt is very low. Some of these people can be helped by therapy. But the painful fact which emerges from the review of the literature on the effectiveness of therapy is that therapy, like medicine, has to be bitter to be helpful. The most striking illustration of this fact comes from research on the use of appetite reducing drugs in weight loss. Even though a combination of drug therapy and behavior therapy has been shown to result in much greater weight loss than behavior therapy alone, behavior therapy patients were much better able to maintain their weight loss than patients who had undergone the combined treatment. It seems important that people are able to attribute their weight loss to their ability to control their eating behavior, a perception which may not develop when weight loss can be attributed to the drug treatment.

Many of the problems which hamper the impact of campaigns that rely on persuasive communications can be circumvented by using strategies aimed at directly changing the rewards and costs associated with a given behavior. Thus, there is evidence that increases in the price of cigarettes or alcoholic beverages reduce the demand for these goods. Similarly, legal restrictions, like increasing the minimal age at which adolescents are allowed to purchase alcohol, or making seatbelt use compulsory, have a positive impact on behavior. The advantage of these legal and economic strategies is that they are useful for both influencing existing habits and preventing new health-impairing habits from developing. The book therefore argues for integrated public health interventions that use both persuasion and changes in incentives to influence health-impairing behavior patterns.

As with our review of health behavior, our discussion of the health consequences of psychosocial stress begins with an assessment of the evidence on the relationship between stress and health. Much of this evidence derives from studies of the relationship between self-reports of cumulative stress events to self-reported health consequences. There are many reasons to doubt these studies, not least the fact that these self-reports are liable to reflect a pervasive mood disposition of negative affectivity. Negative affectivity represents a stable personality disposition to experience negative mood and is closely related to the dimension of neuroticism. While negative affectivity correlates highly with measures of symptom reporting, it seems to be unrelated to objective health indicators such as blood pressure, serum risk factors, or immune system functions. Fortunately, most of the ambiguities involved in using self-report measures of stress can be avoided by studying the health consequences of specific stressful life-events such as researching the health consequences of marital bereavement.

Scientific understanding of the factors which mediate the relationship between stress and health has been greatly improved by the development of cognitive stress theories, as well as by recent advances in physiological research on the impact of stress on the immune system. Another important mediator of the stress health relationship are stress-induced changes in health behavior. Stress has been shown to play an important role in facilitating relapse among people trying to change health-impairing behavior patterns.

The book also reviews both intrapersonal and extrapersonal coping resources such as dispositional optimism and social support, which appear to protect individuals against the deleterious impact of stressful life-events. Since the impact on health of most interpersonal resources seems to be mediated either by cognitive appraisal of the stressful situation or by coping processes, this research raises the possibility that one could direct interventions toward the modification of style of appraisal or coping. Furthermore, since both appraisal and coping are affected by social support, it might also be helpful to provide people with social support, and thereby improve their capacity to deal with stress.

Writing books is one of the unacknowledged sources of psychosocial stress. This book has been no exception. However, the negative effects of the stress and frustration experienced in writing are likely to be counteracted by the many positive experiences. Thus, writing this book has also been fun and a great learning experience. We hope that we have been successful in passing some of the enjoyment and some of the knowledge on to our readers.

Wolfgang Stroebe
Margaret S. Stroebe

ACKNOWLEDGEMENTS

The book profited from the insightful comments and helpful suggestions of a number of colleagues: We would like to express our gratitude to Icek Ajzen, Alice Eagly, and Klaus Jonas who read several chapters and to Bram Buunk who read the whole manuscript. We are particularly indebted to Shelley Taylor for giving us great feedback and encouragement throughout the writing of the manuscript. Although these colleagues helped us to improve the chapters, the final responsibility for the book naturally remains ours.

We would also like to acknowledge the invaluable assistance of Oda von Alvenslebern (Tübingen) and Anna van Fastenhout (Utrecht) in producing the manuscript.

We would finally like to thank Tony Manstead both for his patience and his enthusiastic support.

1 / CHANGING CONCEPTIONS OF HEALTH AND ILLNESS

Good health and a long life are important aims of most persons, but surely no more than a moment's reflection is necessary to convince anyone that they are not the only aim. The economic approach implies that there is an "optimal" expected length of life, where the value in utility of an additional year is less than the utility foregone by using time and other resources to obtain that year. Therefore, a person may be a heavy smoker or so committed to work as to omit all exercise, not necessarily because he is ignorant of the consequences or "incapable" of using the information he possesses, but because the life span forfeited is not worth the cost to him of quitting smoking or working less intensively . . . According to the economic approach therefore, most (if not all!) deaths are to some extent "suicides" in the sense that they could have been postponed if more resources had been invested in prolonging life.

(Becker 1976: 10–11)

The modern increase in life-expectancy

Progress in medical science has been impressive. Knowledge of the body and understanding of disease processes have advanced continuously from the seventeenth century onwards, slowly at first but very rapidly since the turn of the century. This increase in medical knowledge appears to have resulted in a substantial increase in life-expectancy. In 1988, the life-expectancy at birth in the USA averaged 71.3 years for males and 78.3 years for females,

Table 1.1 The 10 leading causes of death in the USA: 1900, 1940 and 1980

Cause of death	1900	1940	1980
Pneumonia and influenza	1	5	6
Tuberculosis (all forms)	2	7	
Diarrhea, enteritis and ulceration of the intestines	3		
Diseases of the heart	4	1	1
Intracranial lesions of vascular origin	5	3	
Nephritis (all forms)	6	4	
All accidents[a]	7	6	4
Cancer[b]	8	2	2
Senility	9		
Diphtheria	10		
Diabetes mellitus		8	7
Motor vehicle accidents		9	
Premature birth		10	
Cardiovascular diseases			3
Chronic, obstructive pulmonary diseases			5
Cirrhosis of the liver			8
Atherosclerosis			9
Suicide			10

[a] This category excludes motor vehicle accidents in the years 1900 and 1940, but includes them in 1980.
[b] This category encompasses cancer and other malignant tumors in the years 1900 and 1940 and changes to malignant neoplasms of all types in 1980.
Source: Matarazzo (1984).

compared with 46.3 years and 48.3 years, respectively, in 1900 (Matarazzo 1984). This increase in longevity has been due mainly to the virtual elimination of those infectious diseases as causes of death that were common at the turn of the century (e.g. pneumonia and influenza, tuberculosis, diphtheria, scarlet fever, measles, typhoid, poliomyelitis). Thus, whereas approximately 40 per cent of all deaths were accounted for by 11 major infections in 1900, only 6 per cent of all deaths were due to these infectious diseases in 1973 (McKinlay & McKinlay 1981). Table 1.1 illustrates this significant shift in the causes of death.

Because this decline in mortality from infectious diseases happened during a time when medical understanding of the causes of these diseases had vastly improved and when vaccines and other chemotherapeutic medical interventions became widely available, it was only plausible to attribute these changes to the efficacy of the new medical measures. However, this may be yet another example of a premature causal inference from purely correlational evidence. After all, during the same period living conditions also improved considerably in most industrialized nations. For large populations in western societies, the problem of malnutrition has been solved and some of the most serious threats to health associated with water and food have been removed by improvements in water supply and sewage disposal.

As can be seen from Figure 1.1, which depicts falls in standardized death rates in the USA for nine common infectious diseases in response to specific medical measures, the declines in mortality took place *before* effective medical interventions became available. McKinlay and McKinlay (1981: 26) concluded from their analysis that "medical measures (both chemotherapeutic and prophylactic) appear to have contributed little to the overall decline in mortality in the United States since about 1900". Similar conclusions were reached by McKeown (1979) on the basis of an even more extensive analysis of data from England and Wales.

Today, the major killers are cardiovascular diseases (i.e. heart disease and stroke) and cancers, with cardiovascular diseases accounting for approximately 40 per cent of deaths in the USA and other industrialized countries. Although deaths from cardiovascular diseases increased during the first half of this century, this pattern has recently begun to reverse. During the last four decades, there has been a small but steady decline in deaths due to heart disease and stroke in the USA and several other industrialized countries (Figure 1.2).

Improvements in medical treatment undoubtedly contributed to this decline, but the significant changes in lifestyle that occurred in the USA during that period were also responsible. Goldman and Cook (1984) even estimated that more than half of the decline in heart disease mortality observed in the USA between 1968 and 1976 was related to changes in lifestyle, specifically the reduction in serum cholesterol levels and cigarette smoking.

Unfortunately, despite advances in medical treatment and significant lifestyle changes, deaths due to cancer – including cancer of the respiratory system – have increased since 1950 in most industrialized countries. However, even though this trend is still

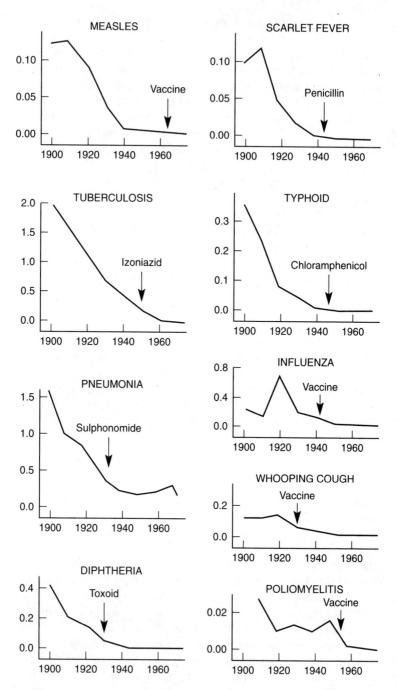

Figure 1.1 The fall in the standardized death rate (per 1000 population) for nine common infectious diseases in relation to specific medical measures in the USA, 1900–1973
Source: McKinlay and McKinlay (1981)

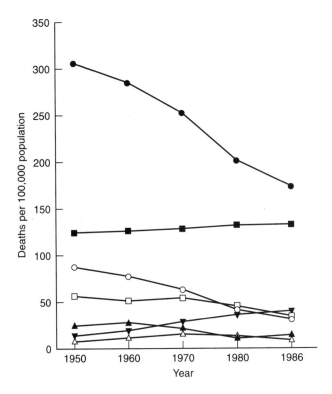

Figure 1.2 Age-adjusted death rates for selected causes of death in the USA, 1950–86. ●, heart disease; ■, malignant neoplasms (all types); ▼, cancer of respiratory system; □, accidents; ○, stroke; ▲, pneumonia and influenza; △, chronic liver disease and cirrhosis of the liver
Source: Adapted from National Center for Health Statistics (1989)

continuing for women in the USA, it has flattened out for men, and in 1985 for the first time in recent years even showed a slight decline (Rothenberg and Koplan 1990).

To summarize, the significant increases in life-expectancy at birth that occurred during this century in most industrialized countries seem to have been only partially attributable to improvements in medical treatment. There is substantial evidence that a purely medical explanation of these changes would be too narrow. Changes in sanitation, nutrition and in lifestyles contributed importantly to the increase in life-expectancy.

The impact of behavior on health

No single set of data can better illustrate the fact that our health is influenced by the way we live than the findings of a prospective study on the health impact of some rather innocuous health behavior, conducted by Belloc, Breslow and their colleagues at the Human Population Laboratory of the California State Department of Public Health (Belloc and Breslow 1972; Belloc 1973; Breslow and Enstrom 1980). In 1965, these researchers asked a representative sample of 6928 residents of Alameda County, California, whether they engaged in the following seven health practices:

1 Sleeping seven to eight hours daily.
2 Eating breakfast almost every day.
3 Never or rarely eating between meals.
4 Currently being at or near prescribed height-adjusted weight.
5 Never smoking cigarettes.
6 Moderate or no use of alcohol.
7 Regular physical activity.

At the time, it was found that good practices were associated with positive health status; those residents who followed all of the good practices were in better health than those who failed to do so, and this association was independent of age, sex and economic status (Belloc and Breslow 1972).

Most striking, however, were the findings of two follow-up studies in which the relationship between these health habits and longevity was explored by using death records. At the first follow-up, conducted $5\frac{1}{2}$ years later, 371 deaths had occurred (Belloc 1973). When the initial health practices in 1965 were then related to subsequent mortality, it was found that the more of these "good" health practices a person engaged in, the greater was the probability that he or she would survive the next $5\frac{1}{2}$ years (Figure 1.3).

These findings were confirmed at a second follow-up investigation conducted $9\frac{1}{2}$ years after the initial inquiry, when again an inverse relationship between health practices and age-adjusted mortality rates was observed (Breslow and Enstrom 1980). Men who followed all seven health practices had a mortality rate which was only 28 per cent of that of men who followed zero to three practices; the comparable rate for women who followed all practices was 43 per cent of those who followed zero to three practices. The authors also observed great stability in the health practices of each individual over the $9\frac{1}{2}$ year period.

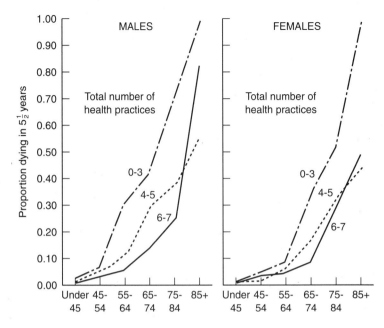

Figure 1.3 Age-specific mortality rates by number of health practices followed by subgroups of males and females
Source: Matarazzo (1984)

Findings such as these (assuming the causal direction is as described here) tend to support Becker's (1976) argument that most deaths are to some extent self-inflicted, at least in the sense that they could have been postponed if people had engaged in "good" health practices, like the ones listed by Belloc and Breslow (1972). The important implication of this research at the individual level is that the responsibility for health does not rest with the medical profession alone. Each of us can have a major impact on the state of our own health. At the institutional level, it emphasizes the potential effectiveness of preventive measures (i.e. primary prevention) that focus on persuading people to adopt good health habits and to change bad ones.

It is important to note, however, that life extension (i.e. mere quantity) is only one of the goals of health promotion, and perhaps not even the most important one. We may have to accept that there is a natural limit to our life-expectancy and that we are unlikely to reach the age of 140, even with the healthiest of lifestyles (Fries

et al. 1989). People are persuaded to engage in a healthy lifestyle
not merely to lengthen their lives but to help them to stay fit
longer and lead an active life right into old age without being
plagued by pain, infirmity and chronic disease. Thus, the second
major goal of health promotion is to increase the quality of life by
delaying the onset of chronic disease and extending the active life-
span (Fries *et al.* 1989).

The impact of stress on health

The concept of stress has become so much part of common culture
that it does not seem to need definition. Reports about health
consequences of everyday stress pervade the advice columns of
popular magazines and even teenagers complain to their teachers
that they are under undue stress due to an overload of homework.
It has become public knowledge that stress, like smoking or drinking too much alcohol, can have adverse effects on physical as well
as mental health.

As we will see in Chapter 7, there is now ample evidence that
psychosocial stress results in health impairment. To some extent,
these health consequences of stressful life-events are mediated by
the same changes in endocrine, immune and autonomic nervous
systems which have been described in the classic work of Selye
(e.g. 1976) on the health impact of physical stressors. However,
the experience of psychosocial stress also causes negative changes
in health behavior that contribute to the stress–illness relationship
(e.g. irregular eating habits, increases in smoking, alcohol consumption and drug intake). Furthermore, stress is often also a
result of people's lifestyles. Thus, research on stress and illness is
closely related to our interest in the impact of behavior on health.

From the biomedical to the biopsychosocial model of disease

That lifestyle factors and psychosocial stress are important determinants of health and illness is difficult to accept within the
framework of the biomedical model, which has been the dominant
model of disease for several centuries (Engel 1977). This model

assumes that for every disease, there exists a primary biological cause that is objectively identifiable. Let us exemplify this approach with statements from a typical medical textbook, *Introduction to Human Disease* (Kent and Hart 1987). According to Kent and Hart, diseases are caused "by injury which may be either external or internal in origin . . . External causes of disease are divided into physical, chemical and microbiologic . . . Internal causes of disease fall into three large categories [vascular, immunologic, metabolic]" (pp. 8–9). Because behavioral factors are not considered to be potential causes of disease, they are also not assessed as part of the process of diagnosis.

By focusing only on the biological causes of illness, the biomedical model disregards the fact that most illnesses are the result of an interaction of social, psychological and biological events. The logical inference of such a biological conception of disease is that physicians need not be concerned with psychosocial issues because they lie outside their responsibility and authority. Thus, the model has little to offer in guiding the kind of preventive efforts that are needed to reduce the incidence of chronic diseases by changing health beliefs, attitudes and behavior.

In recognition of these problems, Engel (1977) proposed an expansion of the biomedical model which incorporates psychosocial factors into the scientific equation. The biopsychosocial model maintains that biological, psychological and social factors are all important determinants of health and illness. According to this approach, medical diagnosis should always consider the interaction of biological, psychological and social factors to assess health and make recommendations for treatment.

Social psychology and health

The growing recognition that lifestyle factors and psychosocial stress contribute substantially to morbidity and mortality from cardiovascular disease, cancer, injuries and other leading causes of death in the industrialized countries was one of the reasons which in the late 1970s led to the development of health psychology as a field which integrates psychological knowledge relevant to the maintenance of health, the prevention of illness and adjustment to illness. Social psychology had, and still has, an important contribution to make to this endeavor, because lifestyles are likely to be determined by health attitudes and health beliefs. Effective prevention has to achieve large-scale changes in lifestyles and such attempts will have to rely on mass communication and thus on the application of the social psychological techniques of attitude and behavior change.

The interest of social psychologists in the study of stress developed more recently, because many of the most stressful life-events (e.g. divorce, bereavement) involve a break-up of social relationships. Furthermore, the health impact of stressful events not only depends on the nature of these events, but also on individuals' ability to cope with a crisis and on the extent to which they receive social support from relatives, friends and other members of their social network. Finally, the impact of stress on health, although to some extent due to the brain's influence on physiological processes such as the body's immune response, is also mediated by the adoption of health-impairing habits such as coping strategies (e.g. smoking, alcohol abuse). Thus, social factors are not only important in determining the stressful nature of many life-events but also as moderators of the stress–health relationship.

Social psychologists have also made important contributions to another major area of health psychology, namely the analysis and improvement of health care systems. This involves issues such as physician–patient relationships, compliance with medical procedures, anxiety as related to medical procedures, and burnout in the helping profession. Although a discussion of social psychological research on these topics would have been highly relevant in the context of this book, we decided against it. Due to limitations of space, any attempt at a complete review of social psychological contributions to health psychology would have had to remain at a superficial level. Instead, we have chosen to present an in-depth analysis of a number of selected areas. The reader interested in social psychological contributions to research into the health care system should consult the excellent overviews provided by Sarafino (1990) and Taylor (1991).

Plan of the book

Why do people engage in health-impairing behavior and how can they be influenced? To answer these questions we need to know and understand the factors and processes that determine the adoption and maintenance of health behavior. Chapter 2 presents the major models of behavior from health and social psychology, thus providing the theoretical framework for the analysis of determinants of health behavior. Chapter 3 discusses strategies of behavior change. We argue that there are basically two stages to the modification of health behavior. Individuals first have to be informed of the health hazards of certain behavior patterns and persuaded to change. This can be achieved by public health interventions such as health education. Because people are often unable to change health-impairing behavior patterns, a second stage may be necessary in which people are taught how to change and how to maintain this change. This second stage usually relies on clinical intervention. Chapter 3 gives an overview of both the public health approach and the methods of clinical intervention.

The next two chapters discuss the major behavioral risk factors that have been linked to health. Chapter 4 focuses on health-impairing behavior such as smoking, alcohol abuse and overeating. These behaviors are addictive in the sense that, once excessive, they are difficult to control. The self-protective behavior covered in Chapter 5, such as eating a healthy diet, safeguarding oneself against accidents and avoiding behavior associated with the risk of AIDS, are in general somewhat more under the volitional control of the individual. In our discussion of these risk factors, we review both the empirical evidence that links these behaviors to negative health consequences and the effectiveness of public health strategies and/or therapy in modifying these behavior patterns.

Chapter 6 discusses causes and consequences of psychosocial stress. Stressful life-events have been related to an increased risk of morbidity and this health impact is not only mediated by the brain's influence on physiological processes, but also by the adoption of health-impairing behaviors as coping strategies.

Chapter 7 reviews personality characteristics and situational factors that serve as interpersonal coping resources and protect individuals from the negative impact of stressful life-events. Our discussion of intrapersonal coping resources focuses on hardiness and dispositional optimism. With regard to extrapersonal coping resources, we mainly review research on the beneficial effects of social support in moderating the impact of stress and discuss psychological mechanisms assumed to mediate this relationship.

In our final outlook presented in Chapter 8, we reflect on the contribution of social psychologists to the public health effort through theories and strategies that help to change health-impairing behavior patterns and reduce psychological stress. We argue for integrated public health interventions that use both persuasion and changes in incentives to influence health-impairing behavior patterns. We also argue for a reorientation of research on behavioral risk factors which focuses less on the extension of total life-expectancy and more on the extension of *active* life-expectancy. It is the reduction of morbidity rather than mortality which makes healthier lifestyles worthwhile for both the individual and society as a whole.

Suggestions for further reading

McKeown, T. (1979). *The role of Medicine*. Oxford: Blackwell. A fascinating analysis of the role of medical measures in the decline of mortality over the last few centuries in England and Wales. It shows that for practically all infectious diseases the major reduction in mortality occurred long before medical measures to cure them had been discovered.

2 / DETERMINANTS OF HEALTH BEHAVIOR: A SOCIAL PSYCHOLOGICAL ANALYSIS

Why do people engage in health-impairing behavior such as smoking or eating a poor diet even if they know that they are damaging their health? Is there any way to influence them to change their behavior? This chapter will present theoretical models from health and social psychology which provide a framework for the analysis of the determinants of health behavior. Knowledge of these determinants will help us to evaluate the potential effectiveness of the strategies of behavior change that will be discussed in the following chapters.

There are several psychological models of behavior which have either been developed specifically to predict health behavior (health belief model; protection motivation theory) or as general models of behavior (theory of reasoned action; theory of planned behavior; the spontaneous processing model). Because these models all agree on the central role of attitudes and beliefs as determinants of behavior, the first part of this chapter will define these central concepts and discuss the relationships between them. The second part of the chapter will then describe and compare these models of behavior. We will also discuss implications of these models for the planning of interventions aimed at changing health behavior.

Attitudes, beliefs and behavior

The concept of attitude

An attitude can be defined as a tendency to evaluate a particular "attitude object" with some degree of favor or disfavor (Eagly and

Chaiken 1993). An attitude object can be any discriminable aspect of the physical or social environment, such as things (cars, drugs), people (doctors, the British), behavior (jogging, drinking alcohol) or even abstract ideas (religion, health). Social psychologists typically divide the evaluative tendencies that reflect an attitude into three classes: cognitive reactions, affective reactions and behavior (e.g. Rosenberg and Hovland 1960; Ajzen 1988; Eagly and Chaiken 1993).

Evaluative responses of the *cognitive* type are thoughts or beliefs about the attitude object. For example, a positive attitude towards jogging might be associated with the belief that jogging helps one to keep one's weight down, increases fitness and decreases high blood pressure. Such beliefs are perceived linkages between the attitude object (i.e. jogging) and various attributes which are positively or negatively valued (i.e. low weight, high blood pressure). Evaluative responses of the *affective* type consist of the emotions that people experience in relation to the attitude object. These evaluative responses also range from extremely positive to extremely negative reactions. For example, these days, many people feel revulsion when they think of fatty foods, whereas the idea of physical exercise makes them feel good. Evaluative responses of the *behavioral* type consist of overt actions towards the attitude object which imply positive or negative evaluations. Thus, people go jogging regularly regardless of weather conditions and ask smokers not to smoke in their presence. Behavioral responses can also consist of behavioral intentions. Thus, the experience of not fitting into ski pants that were too big last season might lead one to form the intention to start a weight loss program next week. Similarly, a smoker who learns that a colleague and fellow smoker has just died from lung cancer might form the intention to stop smoking.

The relationship between attitude and beliefs

It is plausible that people's attitudes should be related to their beliefs about these attitude objects. And indeed, most cognitive theories of attitude share the assumption that the attitude towards some attitude object is a function of the attributes associated with that object and the evaluation of these attributes (e.g. Rosenberg 1960; Fishbein and Ajzen 1975; Sutton 1987). Similarly, a person's attitude towards performing a given behavior is assumed to be a function of the perceived consequences of that behavior and the evaluation of these consequences.

The relationship between attitudes and beliefs can be expressed quantitatively in terms of expectancy-value models (e.g. Fishbein and Ajzen 1975). According to these models, an individual's attitude towards some action depends on the subjective values or utilities attached to the possible outcomes of that action, each weighted by the subjective probabilities that the action will lead to these outcomes. Thus, one's attitude towards personally engaging in physical exercise would be a function of the *perceived likelihood* (i.e. expectancy) with which physical exercise is associated with certain consequences such as low blood pressure or physical fitness, and the *evaluation* (i.e. value, subjective utility) of these consequences. The way such beliefs combine to produce an attitude can be expressed by the following equation:

$$A = \Sigma b_i e_i$$

As can be seen, the subjective probability with which the attitude object is associated with a particular attribute (b) is multiplied by the subjective evaluation (e) of this attribute. The resulting products are summed.

The relationship between attitude and behavior

It would also seem plausible to expect that people who have a positive attitude towards health have healthful lifestyles and refrain from health-impairing behavior such as overeating, drinking too much alcohol, or engaging in unsafe sex. However, the relationship between attitudes and behavior has not proved to be quite so simple. In fact, social psychological research has often failed to find substantial relationships between attitudes and behavior that would seem relevant to these attitudes, particularly when very general attitudes were related to much more specific behavior (for reviews, see Ajzen 1988; Eagly and Chaiken 1993). For example, a study of health attitudes and behavior found that specific health behaviors, such as having regular dental check-ups or eating vitamin supplements, were largely unrelated to general attitudes towards health protection (Ajzen and Timko 1986).

Such findings should not come as a surprise to health psychologists. If different health practices are determined by the same general health attitude, there should be a strong relationship between these practices. People who exercise should also use seatbelts, drink no alcohol and be non-smokers. However, with few exceptions (i.e. people who smoke also over-indulge in alcohol), this does not seem to be the case. Thus, research on the relationship between different health behaviors has found only weak correlations (e.g. Belloc and Breslow 1972; Mechanic 1979).

The lack of correspondence that has frequently been observed in studies of the attitude–behavior relationship does not imply, however, that we should abandon the idea that attitudes are predictors or determinants of behavior. Since the early 1970s, social psychologists have studied the conditions under which measures of attitude predict behavior. In their extensive analyses of attitude–behavior research, Ajzen and Fishbein (1975, 1977) identified two conditions which were usually fulfilled by those studies that found attitude strongly related to behavior – a relationship between attitude and behavior was most likely to emerge if both attitude and behavior had been assessed by measures which were (a) reliable and (b) compatible.

Reliability

Many of the classic studies in the attitude–behavior literature which failed to observe a relationship between attitude and behavior related attitudes to single instances of behavior. As Ajzen and Fishbein (1977) and Epstein (1979) argued, single instances of behavior are determined by a unique set of factors and are thus unreliable measures of behavioral tendencies, that is, the tendency to show a specific behavior over time. For example, even a heavy smoker may refuse a cigarette offered on a particular occasion if he or she has a severe cold or does not like the particular brand of cigarettes. Only when one computes the average behavioral response over repeated occasions does the influence of factors that vary from one occasion to another tend to "cancel out". Thus, when one compares the number of cigarettes smoked on average by a heavy smoker with that smoked by a light smoker or a non-smoker, the cigarette consumption of the heavy smoker is likely to be higher. That aggregation across multiple instances of the same behavior will increase the measure's temporal stability has been amply demonstrated (e.g. Epstein 1979).

Unfortunately, this kind of aggregation does not solve the issue of attitude–behavior consistency in the health area. Health psychologists typically enquire about the frequency with which a set of individuals engage in health-related behavior during a particular period of time. For example, Belloc and Breslow (1972) asked their subjects whether they often, sometimes or never engaged in active sports, or how often they drank alcohol, and so on. Subjects are thus required to provide summary statements about their typical behavior. If these statements are truthful, they are based on a person's recall of repeated instances of performing a given class of behavior like "engaging in active sports" or "drinking alcohol" at different times and in different contexts. Therefore, such estimates reflect *aggregates* across multiple instances of the same behavior and should be reasonably reliable measures of behavioral tendencies. And yet, they have often been found to show rather low correlations with global health attitudes (Ajzen and Timko 1986).

Compatibility

The use of reliable measures is a necessary but not a sufficient condition to achieve high correlations between measures of attitudes and behavior. To ensure a strong relation between measures of attitudes and behavior, these measures not only need to be reliable but also compatible. Measures of attitude and behavior are compatible if both are assessed at the same level of generality. Ajzen and Fishbein (1977) developed some criteria which help to evaluate the degree of compatibility between measures of attitude and behavior. Every instance of behavior involves four specific elements: (1) a specific action, (2) performed with respect to a given target, (3) in a given context and (4) at a given point in time. The principle of compatibility specifies that measures of attitude and behavior are compatible to the extent that their target, action, context and time elements are assessed at identical levels of generality or specificity (Ajzen 1988).

For example, a person's attitude towards a "healthful lifestyle" only specifies the target, but leaves action, context and time elements unspecified. A healthful lifestyle comprises numerous health practices that can be performed in many different contexts at many different times. A behavioral measure that would be compatible with this global attitude would have to aggregate a wide range of health behaviors across different contexts and times.

Consistent with this assumption, Ajzen and Timko (1986) reported that a measure of global attitudes towards health maintenance, which did not correlate significantly with the self-reported frequency with which subjects performed *specific* health-protecting behaviors, showed a substantial correlation with a behavioral index that aggregated the performance of a wide variety of different health-protecting behaviors. These behaviors related to different aspects of health and had been performed in a wide variety of contexts and times.

On the other hand, if we are interested in predicting *specific* behavior, then an attitude measure would be compatible if it assessed the attitude towards performing the specific behavior. Thus, Ajzen and Timko (1986) were able to predict specific health behaviors from equally specific attitudes towards these behaviors. For example, the reported frequency with which subjects' had "regular dental check-ups" correlated 0.46 with subjects' attitudes "towards having regular dental check-ups".

The principle of compatibility has implications for strategies of attitude and behavior change. As with prediction, compatibility should be observed in attempts to change behavior. Thus, mass media campaigns designed to change some specific health behavior should use arguments mainly aimed at changing beliefs relating to that *specific* behavior rather than focusing on more general health concerns. For example, to persuade people to lower the cholesterol content of their diet, it would not be very effective merely to point out that coronary heart disease is the major killer and/or that high cholesterol levels are bad for one's heart. To influence diets one would have to argue that very specific changes in one's diet, such as eating less animal fats and less red meat, would have a positive impact on blood cholesterol levels and that the reduction in serum cholesterol should in turn reduce the risk of developing coronary heart disease.

Models of behavior

The assumption that attitudes and beliefs are major determinants of behavior is shared by five major models of behavior, from each of which predictions about health behavior can be made. These models are the health belief model, protection motivation theory, theory of reasoned action, theory of planned behavior and the spontaneous processing model. With the exception of the spontaneous processing model, these theories belong to the family of expectancy-value models. As we explained earlier, expectancy-value models make the assumption that decisions between different courses of action are based on two types of cognition: (1) subjective probabilities that a given action will lead to a set of expected outcomes, and (2) evaluation of action outcomes. Individuals will choose among various alternative courses of action that action which will be most likely to lead to positive consequences or avoid negative consequences. The models described in this section elaborate the basic model by specifying the *types* of beliefs and attitudes which should be used in predicting a particular class of behavior and/or by incorporating *additional* variables such as subjective norms or perceived control to predict behavior. By examining the extent to which various factors suggested by these models affect behavior, empirical studies of these models are not only informative with regard to our ability to predict behavior in a particular domain, they also provide important insights into ways of influencing that behavior. For example, if behavior in a given domain is found to be only weakly related to attitudes but strongly related to subjective norms, attempts at changing that behavior should focus on changing subjective norms rather than attitudes.

The health belief model

The health belief model was originally developed by social psychologists in the US Public Health Service in an attempt to understand why people failed to make use of disease prevention or screening tests for the early detection of diseases not associated with clear-cut symptoms, at least in the early stages. Later, the model was also applied to patients' responses to symptoms and compliance with or adherence to prescribed medical regimens. In the course of these applications, the model was considerably expanded (for reviews, see Rosenstock 1974; Wallston and Wallston 1981; Janz and Becker 1984).

The model
The health belief model assumes that the likelihood that an individual engages in a given health behavior will be a function (a) of the extent to which a person believes that he or she is personally

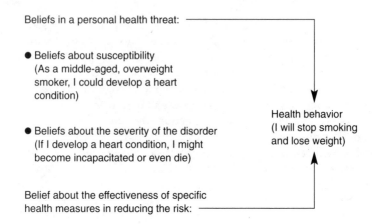

Figure 2.1 The health belief model applied to the health behaviors of giving up smoking and losing weight

susceptible to the particular illness, and (b) of his or her perceptions of the *severity* of the consequences of getting the disease. Susceptibility and severity jointly determine the *perceived-threat* of the disease, sometimes also referred to as vulnerability (see Figure 2.1). For example, a middle-aged male smoker who is overweight and who has high blood pressure, might know that he is at great risk of cardiovascular disease (perceived susceptibility) and that he could be completely incapacitated or even die from such a condition (perceived severity).

Given some threat of the disease, the likelihood of engaging in a particular health behavior will further depend on the extent to which the individual believes that the action yields *benefits* that outweigh the *barriers* associated with the action, such as the costs, inconvenience or pain. For example, whether the overweight smoker will decide to stop smoking, reduce his weight, and/or go jogging will depend upon his estimate of whether the benefits to his health associated with these actions would really outweigh the costs in terms of loss of pleasure and the effort of going jogging.

Rosenstock (1974) further suggested that a *cue to action* might be necessary to trigger appropriate health behavior. This could be an internal cue like a bodily symptom, or an external cue such as a mass media campaign, medical advice, or the death of a colleague similar in age and lifestyle. For example, our middle-aged man might be triggered into health-protecting action if he suddenly experienced strange chest pains or his doctor advised him to change his lifestyle.

The relation between the variables of the health belief model has never been formalized or even explicitly spelled out, but on the basis of discussions of the model and the way researchers using the model analysed their data, Seibold and Roper (1979) suggested the following mathematical representation:

$$LA(f)PV_{w_1} + PS_{w_2} + (PB - PC)_{w_3}$$

where LA, the likelihood of a person taking preventive action, is a function (f) of the following variables: PV = perceived vulnerability to the disease, PS = perceived severity of the consequences associated with the disease, PB = perceived benefits from enacting the positive health behavior, and PC = the costs associated with the behavior; w_1, w_2 and w_3 reflect the empirically determined weights which specify the relationship between each component and the criterion, LA.

The additive combination of the variables of the health belief model implies that the influence of each of the variables on health behavior is not moderated by any of the other factors. For example, the assumption that the threat of a disease is a function of the *sum* of (a) the perceived susceptibility of contracting a disease and (b) the perceived severity of the disease, implies that there is a moderate threat as long as one of these two variables is high, even if the other approaches zero. In contrast, intuition would tell us that the perceived threat of an illness would be very low if either of the two factors had a value of zero. For example, there may be many deadly diseases in the world (high severity) which do not worry us, because there is not the slightest chance that we could contract them (low susceptibility). With other diseases, the chance of contracting them might be high, but the consequences might be so minor that we would not really take preventive action.

The type of relationship in which the impact of each of the factors on health behavior is dependent on the level of the other factor would be better represented by a model using some kind of multiplicative combination of the components. However, even though a multiplicative combination of the components is intuitively more plausible than the additive combination, researchers in the health area have often failed to demonstrate the multiplicative combination between severity and probability of threat (e.g. Rogers and Mewborn 1976; for a review, see Jonas 1993). Jonas (1993) argued that the failure to support a multiplicative model may be due to the fact that people are unable to perform the kind of trade-offs between expectancies and valences that are required by a multiplicative combination of the two variables. He presented empirical findings which support this assumption.

According to the health belief model, there can be many reasons why individuals do not change their health behavior even if their actual vulnerability is high. There is evidence of a pervasive tendency for people to underestimate their own health risks compared with those of others (Weinstein 1987). Thus, even if people accept that eating a fatty diet increases the risk of heart disease, they might feel protected by a particularly hardy constitution. But even if individuals perceive a threat realistically, they are unlikely to engage in health-protecting measures if they doubt their effectiveness or if they feel that the effort is just too great to make it worthwhile. Thus, any media campaign aimed at modifying health behavior should contain arguments which persuade them (a) that serious health consequences are likely to occur, unless they change certain aspects of their lifestyle, *and* (b) that the adoption of specific health behaviors would considerably reduce this risk.

Empirical evaluation of the model
Janz and Becker (1984) reviewed 46 studies based on the health belief model, of which 18 used prospective and 28 retrospective designs. In order to assess support for the model, they constructed a "significance ratio" for each dimension, which divided the number of positive, statistically significant findings for a given dimension of the model by the total number of studies reporting significance

levels for this dimension. The results were as follows: barriers (89 per cent), susceptibility (81 per cent), benefits (78 per cent) and severity (65 per cent). The authors interpret these results as providing substantial support for the model.

However, the fact that the association between two variables is statistically significant is not very informative concerning the strength of the relationship. To evaluate the strength of an association we would need information about "effect sizes", which would allow us to estimate the variance in health behavior that is accounted for by the various components of the model either separately or jointly. During the last decade, relevant procedures have been developed, which are called *meta-analysis*. Meta-analysis allows one to quantify study outcomes of a comprehensive sample of studies on a given topic in terms of a common metric (effect sizes), which allow comparisons across studies and the examination of overall outcomes of the findings of all the studies combined (e.g. Rosenthal 1991). Although meta-analyses have been conducted in some of the areas to be discussed later, to our knowledge no meta-analysis is available on the health belief model.

Implications for the planning of interventions
The implications of the health belief model for interventions aimed at influencing some domain of health behavior are illustrated by the findings of a study which applied the model to condom use among teenagers (Abraham *et al.* 1992). This study of more than 300 sexually active Scottish teenagers, which investigated the relation between the various components of the health belief model and intention to carry and use condoms, found perceived severity of HIV infection, perceived vulnerability to HIV infection and perceived effectiveness of condom use only weakly related to intention. In contrast, perceived barriers to condom use (e.g. beliefs concerning pleasure reduction, awkwardness of use, and one's partner's likely response to suggested use) were found to be substantially related to intentions to carry and use condoms. These findings suggest that instead of emphasizing young people's vulnerability to infection, the severity of infection and condom effectiveness, as had been done in most previous interventions, it might be more effective to focus on social acceptability barriers in future interventions.

Protection motivation theory

The original model

Although protection motivation theory has mainly been tested in the context of fear-arousing communications, the original version of the theory (e.g. Rogers and Mewborn 1976) constituted an attempt to specify the algebraic relationship between some of the components of the health belief model. According to the theory, protection motivation (that is, the motivation to engage in some kind of health-protecting behavior) depends on three factors: (1) the perceived severity of the noxious event; (2) the perceived probability of the event's occurrence or perceived susceptibility; and (3) the efficacy of the recommended response in averting the noxious event. The model does not include the costs of the recommended response as a variable.

According to this model, the response of a smoker exposed to a campaign that emphasizes the causal role of smoking in the development of lung cancer will depend on his answer to the following questions: "How bad is it to have lung cancer?" "How likely is it that I will get lung cancer?" "How much would giving up smoking reduce my risk of getting lung cancer?" The model assumes that the three factors combine multiplicatively to determine the intensity of protection motivation. More specifically, the intensity of protection motivation is assumed to be a monotonically increasing function of the algebraic product of these three variables.

An empirical test of the original model

Rogers and Mewborn (1976) tested the predictions of protection motivation theory in a series of three experiments, which used fear appeals on the topics of smoking, traffic safety and venereal diseases. In these experiments, fear-arousing communications manipulated each of the three crucial variables of theory at two levels: high *vs* low noxiousness of the depicted event; high *vs* low probability of that event's occurrence; and high *vs* low efficacy of the recommended coping response. The results differed across the three studies and did not provide clear support for the model. In particular, in none of the three experiments was there any evidence of the three-way interaction (perceived susceptibility × perceived severity × perceived efficacy of coping) that would be expected on the basis of the multiplicative combination of the three factors of the model.

As Sutton (1982) pointed out, the failure of the study of Rogers and Mewborn (1976) to support the model could have been due to the fact that perceived efficacy and susceptibility are not independent of each other, as the model assumes. The recommended action is perceived as effective to the extent that it is thought to reduce the risk of occurrence of the noxious event. Therefore, perceived efficacy can never be greater than perceived susceptibility. This, he argued, leads to inconsistencies in some conditions of the experiment. For example, under conditions of *high effectiveness* and *low vulnerability*, subjects are told that taking protective actions will considerably reduce their risk of contracting a particular disease, even though they have already been informed that there is little chance of them getting it. This kind of inconsistency may account for the fact that experimental tests failed to find many of the interactive effects predicted by the model.

The revised model

In a revision of protection motivation theory, Rogers (1983; Rippetoe and Rogers 1987) abandoned the notion that the various factors combine multiplicatively and also expanded the theory by including additional determinants of protection motivation. Probably the most important variable to be added was *self-efficacy*. The concept of self-efficacy refers to a person's belief that he or she is able to perform a particular action (Bandura 1986). Because people might not be motivated to stop smoking or give up alcohol despite a negative attitude towards these behaviors (because they are addicted or too weak to do so), the inclusion of self-efficacy in a model of health protective behavior should improve predictions. The revision also incorporated the health belief model's perceived barrier construct (labelled "response costs") and added a related one, the rewards associated with "maladaptive" responses (e.g. the enjoyment of continuing to drink or smoke, the time and energy saved by not having health check-ups).

The revised model assumes that the motivation to protect oneself from danger is a positive linear function of four beliefs: (1) the threat is severe, (2) one is personally vulnerable, (3) one has the ability to perform the coping response, and (4) the coping response is effective in reducing the threat. The motivation to perform the adaptive response is negatively influenced by the costs of that response and by potential rewards associated with maladaptive responses.

More specifically, Rogers divides these six variables into two classes – threat appraisal and coping appraisal. As shown in Figure 2.2, each of these classes is further divided into two components (e.g. extrinsic/intrinsic rewards for the maladaptive response and vulnerability/severity in the case of threat appraisal). Rogers assumes that the variables within each of these two classes should exert an additive effect on protection motivation and intention. Across the threat appraisal and coping appraisal classes, however, interaction effects are postulated. Research supporting these assumptions has been reviewed by Rogers (1983).

Implications for interventions

These assumptions have important implications for the planning of interventions. For example, if self-efficacy for a given behavior domain has been found to be relatively high in a target population (i.e. if most individuals feel competent to engage in a recommended health-protecting action), the provision of information which increases vulnerability or severity should increase protection motivation and thus intention to act. Under these conditions, individuals should be more likely to take action the greater they perceive their individual risk. When self-efficacy is low, however – that is, when most individuals feel that they are unable to engage in a given action (e.g. dieting to lose weight) – increases in vulnerability should not result in increments in intentions. Under the latter conditions, rather than emphasizing risk, it might be more effective to provide individuals with information which increases their self-efficacy.

Conclusions

Both the health belief model and protection motivation theory have generated a great deal of research in the health area. During the last few decades, however, a number of more general models of behavior have been developed which have also been applied to the health area. Obviously, it is not very economic to continue to entertain specific theories of health behavior unless the predictive success of these models is greater than that of general models of behavior. Although we would argue that the general models of behavior to be presented in the following sections of this chapter have been more successful in predicting behavior than the two theories of health behavior just described, it is difficult to validate

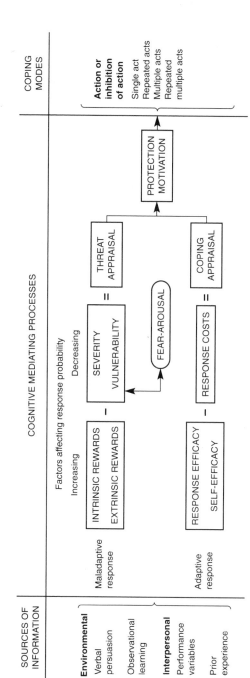

Figure 2.2 Schema of protection motivation theory
Source: Rippetoe and Rogers (1987)

this impression empirically, due to a lack of studies comparing these various models.

The theory of reasoned action

One of the more general social psychological models of behavior, namely the theory of reasoned action (e.g. Fishbein and Ajzen 1975), has been tested extensively and has been successful in predicting a wide range of behaviors (for reviews, see Ajzen 1988; Eagly and Chaiken 1993).

The model
The theory of reasoned action predicts behavioral intention and assumes that behavior is a *function* of the intention to perform that behavior. A behavioral intention is determined by one's attitude towards performing the behavior and by subjective norms. Thus people's intentions to stop smoking will depend on their attitude towards stopping to smoke, which in turn will be the result of their beliefs about the consequences of stopping to smoke (Figure 2.3). As we outlined earlier, a person's attitude towards giving up smoking will be a function of the perceived likelihood that cessation is associated with certain consequences, such as being healthier and fitter or reducing the risk of developing heart problems or lung cancer.

It is important to note that the perceived consequences of smoking should affect intentions to stop only if individuals believe that the negative consequences of continuing to smoke are likely to happen to *them*. If a smoker is convinced that although smoking is generally unhealthy, he or she is unlikely to suffer any negative consequences (e.g. due to a particular hardiness that runs in the family), these general beliefs will not affect the individual's attitude towards performing that behavior.

Subjective norms are beliefs about how people who are important to us expect us to behave. For example, a woman might believe that her husband does not want her to indulge in dangerous sports or that he would like her to lose some weight. However, whether such normative beliefs influence intentions will also depend on one's willingness to comply with this norm. Thus, subjective norms are normative beliefs weighted by motivation to comply. The model quantifies these normative beliefs by multiplying

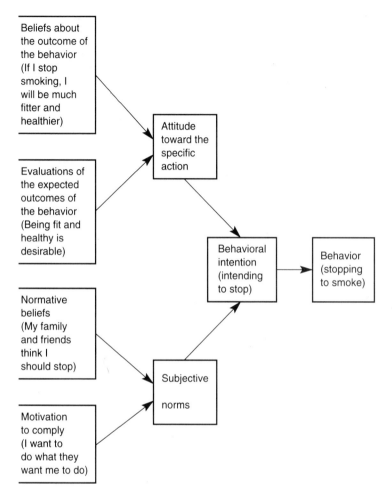

Figure 2.3 The theory of reasoned action applied to the decision to give up smoking

the subjective likelihood that a particular other (the referent) thinks the person should perform the behavior multiplied by the person's motivation to comply with that referent's expectation. These products are analogous to the expectancy × value products computed for behavioral beliefs and are also summed over various salient referent persons. Because both attitudes and normative beliefs reflect expectations regarding the consequences of a given behavior weighted by the valence of these consequences, the model of reasoned action also belongs to the class of expectancy-value models.

Implications for interventions

According to the model, the effectiveness of strategies aimed at modifying health behavior depends on the success in changing attitudes towards the specific behavior and relevant subjective norms. One way to modify attitudes is to persuade individuals that their present behavior exposes them to the risk of negative health consequences which could be avoided by a change in behavior. Attitudes can also be changed by modifying the environment so as to increase the costs of the health-impairing behavior (e.g. increases in the price of tobacco; restrictions on the sale of alcoholic beverages; introduction of legal sanctions for not using seatbelts). However, increasing the costs of health-impairing behavior will affect behavior only if the person is aware of these changes and if the costs are sufficiently high to outweigh the benefits. For example, the introduction of financial sanctions for failing to use seatbelts will influence the relevant behavior only if the person realizes that the law has been changed, thinks that there is a good chance of getting caught if he or she does not comply, and feels that the penalty is large enough to outweigh the expected discomfort of wearing belts.

Whether one should focus more on attitudes or subjective norms in designing a campaign to influence a specific behavior will depend on the relative weight which the two components of the model have in determining the behavior in question. For example, subjective norms seem to be *less* important than attitudes for women's choice between breast- versus bottle-feeding (Manstead *et al.* 1983). On the other hand, a woman's decision to have an abortion (Smetana and Adler 1980) or a couple's decision to have another child (Vinokur-Kaplan 1978) have been found to be *more* strongly affected by perceived social pressure than by personal attitudes.

Empirical evaluation of the model

The model of reasoned action has been successful in predicting a wide range of behaviors. It has been applied to blood donation, family planning, eating at fast-food restaurants, smoking marijuana, mothers' infant feeding practices, dental hygiene behavior and having an abortion (for a review, see Eagly and Chaiken 1993). In an extensive meta-analysis of research on the model based on 113 articles, Van den Putte (1991) reported the following estimates of the various relations of the model based on 150 groups of respondents: The average multiple correlation for predicting intention from attitudes and subjective norms was 0.68, and the average correlation for predicting behavior from intention was 0.62. Thus, attitudes and subjective norms accounted for approximately 46 per cent of the variance in intentions and for 38 per cent of the variance in behavior. Van den Putte also found that the relation between intention and attitude was stronger than the relation between intention and subjective norms.

Omissions from the model

Despite the success in predicting intention and behavior, the model has been criticized by researchers who have argued that intentions and actions are affected by a number of factors which are not included in the model of reasoned action. The most interesting of these additional determinants in the context of a discussion of health behavior is past behavior. In a test of the theory of reasoned action that used self-reported consumption of alcohol, marijuana and hard drugs as dependent measures, Bentler and Speckart (1979) found that reported past behavior added to the prediction of future behavior even when intention was statistically controlled. This finding has been replicated in a number of other studies for exercise (Bentler and Speckart 1981), condom use (de Wit *et al.* 1990; Schaalma *et al.* 1993) and seatbelt use (Sutton and Hallett 1989). In these later studies, multiple-regression analyses showed that the prediction of behavior was improved by the addition of past behavior over and above the prediction achieved on the basis of intention.

The problem of volitional control

The finding that measures of past behavior add to the prediction of future behavior even when intentions are statistically controlled, could represent the impact of any number of factors that influence behavior but which are not taken into account by the theory of reasoned action. In interpreting these findings, we have to remember that the theory of reasoned action offers a theoretical account of the factors that determine intentions. Intentions only reflect the motivation to act. Execution of an action not only depends on motivation but also on whether the behavior is under

the volitional control of the individual. A behavior is under volitional control if the individual can decide at will whether or not
to perform it. Thus, past behavior might reflect the influence of
factors that are not under the volitional control of the individual.
Considering the type of behavior used in studies that found an
independent influence of past behavior on future behavior, it would
seem plausible that two major factors reflected by past behavior
are *habit* and *lack of control*.

Some actions may have become so routinized and habitual that
people perform them without even thinking about them. For example, smokers might light a cigarette or a pipe without intending
to do so or even realizing that they are doing it. Because past
behavior would have also been influenced by their habit, using
past behavior to predict future behavior would then improve predictions even when intentions are statistically controlled.

Motivational problems could also be responsible for the finding
that past behavior improves the prediction of future actions. Particularly in the health area, there are abundant examples of behavior
that are only under very incomplete voluntary control of the individual. For example, people who try to give up smoking rarely
manage to do so at their first attempt, and people who try to lose
weight often weaken at mealtimes or when they walk by a bakery
or a food store. The fact that people often experience difficulties
in controlling their behavior could in part be responsible for the
finding that past behavior improves prediction of future behavior,
particularly in research on the use of drugs, smoking or alcohol
consumption.

There are many factors which could lower the control individuals have over their actions. As Liska (1984: 63) pointed out in an
influential critique of the theory of reasoned action, the restriction
of the Fishbein–Ajzen model to behavior that is under volitional
control also excludes behavior that requires "skills, abilities, opportunities and the cooperation of others". According to this view,
the great majority of studies that have supported the theory of
reasoned action have involved relatively simple behaviors that do
not require much in the way of resources and skills (Eagly and
Chaiken 1993).

Fishbein and Ajzen (1975) were not unaware of this issue, but
they argued that people would take the need for resources or
others' cooperation into account in forming their intentions.
Changes in resources will then result in changes in intention. For

example, if somebody who intended to play tennis with a friend on Monday evening learns that their friend has fallen ill, that person is likely to change his or her intention. Such unexpected changes in external conditions are one of the reasons why intentions predict behavior better the shorter the time-lag between the assessment of intentions and behavior.

Although this position is reasonable, the restriction of the model of reasoned action to behaviors that are under complete volitional control seriously limits the applicability of the model. Closer inspection reveals that very few behaviors are under the complete volitional control of an individual. Even the execution of such simple actions as brushing one's teeth depends on the availability of one's toothbrush and toothpaste.

The theory of planned behavior

The model

This type of reasoning has led Ajzen to modify the theory of reasoned action and to develop the theory of planned behavior (Ajzen 1988, 1991). The model of planned behavior incorporates perceived control over the behavior to be predicted as an additional predictor. Perceived controllability of a behavior can be assessed directly by asking subjects to what extent performing a given behavior was under their control. The concept is thus very similar to the construct of self-efficacy, which reflects people's judgments of their capabilities to execute certain courses of action required to attain intended levels of performance (Bandura 1986). The model of planned behavior assumes that perceived control can affect behavior indirectly through intentions. Under certain conditions, it can also have a direct effect on behavior that is not mediated by intentions (Figure 2.4).

The assumption that perceived control affects intentions is consistent with expectancy-value theories of motivation. People who lack the ability or the opportunity to achieve some goal will adjust their intentions accordingly, because intentions are partly determined by people's perception of the probability that a goal can be reached by them. For example, students who have learned from past performance that they lack the ability to achieve the kind of outstanding grades in their courses that they had hoped for, are

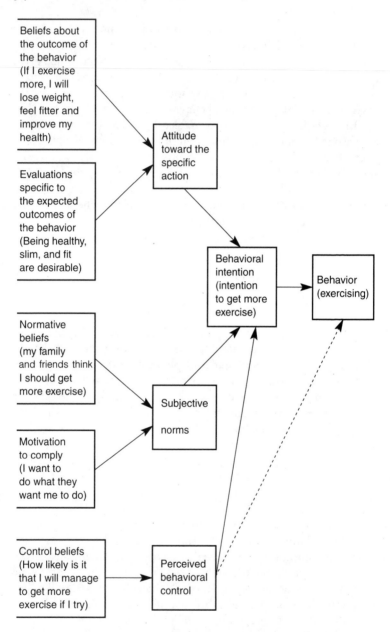

Figure 2.4 The theory of planned behavior applied to the intention to engage in physical exercise

likely to adjust their intentions and aim for lower but more realistic grades.

The direct relationship between perceived control and behavior which is not mediated by intentions (indicated by the broken line in Figure 2.4) is intuitively less plausible, but can be illustrated by the following example. A businesswoman who likes to jog every evening may also know that on many evenings she has to entertain out-of-town customers and that their visits will prevent her from exercising. Thus, although she would indicate that she has every intention to jog daily, she would also have to admit that her time is not her own. Her *realistic* rating of the extent to which she has control over whether or not she jogs every evening will therefore be an additional predictor of her jogging that is not mediated by her intentions.

It is important to note that the direct link of perceived control to behavior has a somewhat different theoretical status from the link that is mediated by intention. Whereas perceived control has a causal influence on intentions (e.g. the authors' knowledge of their lack of will-power has prevented them from ever forming the intention to jog), it is not the perceived but the *actual* lack of control which *causally* influences behavior (via the direct route). Thus, it is not the businesswoman's expectation that out-of-town customers might have to be entertained which prevents her from jogging, but the *actual* visits of customers who have to be entertained.

The latter example can also be used to illustrate that perceived control should only improve the prediction of behavior (which is exclusively based on intentions) if it realistically reflects actual levels of control. Suppose there is an unexpected slump in business and none of the expected out-of-town customers turn up. As a consequence, the woman would have much more control over her jogging than she had anticipated earlier. It is plausible that, under these conditions, perceived control as assessed earlier would not improve predictions of behavior.

In line with this assumption, Ajzen and Madden (1986) found in a study of grades based on repeated examinations, that the direct link between perceived control and behavior only emerged when perceived control was assessed *after* students had taken one of the exams. Supposedly, their estimate of their own control over grades had become more realistic after they had taken their first test.

Determinants of perceived control
The factors that influence perceived control can either be internal or external to the individual (Ajzen 1988). Examples of internal factors are information, skills, abilities, and also urges and compulsions. Our control over health behavior is often threatened by those internal factors that are collectively referred to as "willpower". Thus, despite the firm intention to visit a doctor or to lose weight, a person with medical or weight problems may know from past experience that he or she is unlikely to execute these intentions. Examples of external factors are opportunity and dependence on others (Ajzen 1988). For example, we know that we can only go cross-country skiing tomorrow if the snow does not melt and if our boss allows us to leave the office on time.

Another important distinction that should be considered in discussing perceived control is that between efficacy expectancy and outcome expectancy. An *efficacy* expectancy is the expectation that, if one tried to perform a certain behavior, one would be able to do it. For example, an obese individual might be fairly confident that he or she could substantially reduce daily calorie consumption. Nevertheless, as we will find out later, a reduction in calorie intake might not necessarily result in substantial weight loss. Thus, whereas the perceived likelihood that one is able to reduce one's calorie intake is an efficacy expectancy, the expectation that this reduction will actually result in substantial weight loss is an *outcome* expectancy. The concept of perceived control as used by Ajzen refers to both outcome expectancy and efficacy expectancy.

Empirical evaluation of the model
The model of planned behavior has been applied to a variety of behaviors, ranging from academic grades to shop-lifting (for a review, see Ajzen 1991). The first published test of the model was a study of weight loss (Schifter and Ajzen 1985). Female college students were asked at the beginning of the study to express their attitudes, subjective norms, perceived control and intentions with respect to losing weight during a 6 week period. In addition, the extent to which the participants had made detailed weight reduction plans was assessed, as were a number of general attitudes and personality factors. Consistent with the theory, the intention to lose weight was predicted quite accurately on the basis of attitudes, subjective norms and perceived control. However, perceived control

and intentions were only moderately successful in predicting the amount of weight that the participants actually lost during the 6 weeks (i.e. an outcome), with perceived control being the better predictor. As expected, there was also an interaction between perceived control and intention on weight reduction – a strong intention to lose weight increased weight reduction only for those participants who believed that they would be able to control their calorie intake, if they wanted to. Those subjects who had made a detailed plan at the beginning of the period also tended to lose more weight.

Since then, more than a dozen empirical tests have been published (Ajzen 1991). The results of these studies tend to support the central predictions of the model of planned behavior. Thus, in most studies, the incorporation of perceived control improved the prediction of both intentions and behavior. In his review, Ajzen (1991) reports an average multiple correlation of 0.71 for the prediction of intentions and of 0.51 for behavior. In nearly all the studies reviewed by Ajzen (1991), the inclusion of perceived control in the regression equation resulted in a significant improvement in the prediction of behavior. This finding supports the assumption that, unless a given behavior is under the complete volitional control of an individual, predictions of behavior from the model of planned behavior are superior to those based on the theory of reasoned action.

Implications for interventions
The assumption that the intention to engage in a specific health-protecting behavior is mainly determined by attitudes towards that behavior, by relevant subjective norms and by perceived control, has important implications for interventions aimed at influencing that behavior. Such interventions should only be effective if they influence relevant attitudes, norms and control perceptions. Support for this assumption comes from an experimental study of the effectiveness of a health education program on AIDS developed by Dutch Educational Television (de Wit *et al.* 1990). Two groups of male and female students attending secondary schools were assessed at two points in time, using a questionnaire which measured AIDS-relevant knowledge as well as attitudes towards condom use, perceived norms regarding condom use, perceived control over condom use, and intention to use condoms. In the time between the two assessments, half the subjects were exposed to the

health education program on AIDS, whereas the other half were not exposed to the information.

The students reported that they learned a great deal of new information from the program. Consistent with these self-reports, the intervention group showed a significant increase in relevant knowledge. However, despite its impact on AIDS knowledge, the intervention did not influence intentions to use condoms. Intentions were solely determined by attitudes towards condom use, perceived norms and perceived effectiveness. This finding is in line with the results of other studies indicating that neither knowledge nor perceived susceptibility seem to be related to behavioral risk reduction regarding HIV infection (e.g. Richard and van der Pligt 1991; Abraham *et al.* 1992). The obvious implication from such findings is that future AIDS campaigns should give less emphasis to AIDS knowledge and focus more on attitudes towards condom use, subjective norms and perceived effectiveness.

Beyond reasons and plans: The spontaneous processing model

The models of behavior discussed in this chapter conceive of people as fairly rational decision makers who tend to deliberate about future actions to form a behavioral intention. Even though none of these models assumes that individuals have to weigh all the consequences of the behavioral alternatives at each behavioral opportunity, the fact that they all more or less imply that behavior is mediated by intentions suggests that behavior involves at least a minimum of cognitive deliberations.

Fazio (1990) has recently suggested that the central aspects of such a deliberative process – the formation and retrieval of attitudes toward a behavior or of a behavioral intention – occur only when individuals are both able and willing to consciously attend to and think about future actions. People are more likely to expend cognitive effort on their actions if the behavioral outcomes are important to them and if they have the time and the peace of mind to deliberate. When behavioral outcomes are not very important or when individuals have little opportunity for deliberation, attitudes might affect behavior through a *spontaneous* processing mode. A related conceptualization has been suggested by Kruglanski (1989).

The model

Fazio and his colleagues have suggested that such spontaneous behaviors are influenced by attitudes toward objects or targets rather than by attitudes toward behavior (Fazio 1986, 1990). According to the spontaneous processing model, the attitude-to-behavior sequence is initiated when attitudes are accessed from memory by the presentation of cues related to the attitude objects. This activation process is assumed to be automatic in the sense that it is relatively effortless and not mediated by active attention or conscious deliberation (Eagly and Chaiken 1993). The likelihood of such automatic activation of the attitude upon mere observation of the attitude object is a function of the *accessibility* of the attitude. The accessibility or ease of recall of an attitude will depend on the strength of the association that exists in memory between the attitude object and the individual's evaluation of the object. Only if the evaluation is strongly associated with the object is it likely that the evaluation will be activated spontaneously upon observation of the attitude object. If the association between object and evaluation is weak, the automatic attitude-to-behavior sequence will not occur.

After a strong attitude has been accessed automatically, it is assumed to exert a selective influence on the person's perception of the attitude object. This selectivity means that the qualities of the attitude object are perceived as congruent with one's attitude, a congruence that might be achieved by considerable distortion of reality. When positive attitudes are activated, positive qualities are attributed to the attitude object, whereas negative qualities are attributed upon the activation of a negative attribute. Thus, although seeing somebody work out (and sweat) vigorously might activate positive thoughts of health and fun in aerobics fanatics, it might activate feelings of exhaustion and distaste among the non-energetic. These perceptions of the attitude object "comprise at least part of the individual's definition of the event" (Fazio 1986: 213). Normative factors (e.g. expectations of others, rules about correct behavior) can also influence the definition of the event and thus also affect behavior. The model is depicted in Figure 2.5.

Empirical evaluation of the model

The research of Fazio and his colleagues has in the main addressed two issues: (1) the hypothesis that accessibility of relevant attitudes

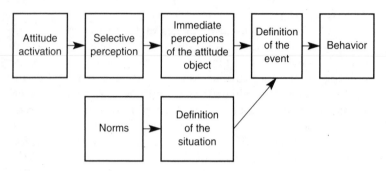

Figure 2.5   The spontaneous processing model
Source: Fazio (1986)

influences the association between attitude and behavior; and (2) the hypothesis that strong attitudes exert a selective influence on perception. Fazio and his colleagues operationalized accessibility of attitudes through the speed with which subjects respond to questions regarding their attitude. This operationalization is based on the assumption that individuals whose attitudes are more readily accessible, will have lower latencies in responding evaluatively to attitude-relevant cues than individuals whose attitudes are less accessible. The assumption derives from an associative model of learning which conceives of attitudes as associations between attitude objects and evaluations.

One major determinant of the accessibility of attitudes according to Fazio and his colleagues is the type of experience on which the attitude is based. They reasoned that attitudes that have been formed on the basis of direct experience rather than indirectly as a result of descriptions of the attitude object would be more accessible. Three types of findings are consistent with the assumption that direct experience with the attitude object increases accessibility of the attitude, which in turn results in higher correlations between attitude and behavior. First, it has been demonstrated that the correlation between attitude and behavior is higher when attitudes have been formed on the basis of direct experience rather than indirectly (e.g. Fazio *et al.* 1982). Second, there is evidence that attitudes which are based on direct experience are responded to with greater speed (e.g. Fazio *et al.* 1982). Third, it has been shown that correlations between attitude and behavior are higher for attitudes which can be activated with short response latencies than for those activated with long response latencies (e.g. Fazio and Williams 1986).

Direct experience is only one of the determinants of accessibility. The association between an evaluation and an object should also be strengthened by the frequency with which the attitude has recently been activated. Consistent with this assumption, Fazio and his colleagues demonstrated that the frequency with which respondents had to express their attitudes was positively related to speed of response and to increases in the correspondence between attitude and behavior (Fazio *et al.* 1982; Fazio and Williams 1986).

A second line of research by Fazio and his colleagues (Fazio and Williams 1986; Houston and Fazio 1989) addressed the proposition that attitudes which are highly accessible have a selective effect on perception. For example, Fazio and Williams (1986) assessed the speed with which respondents answered questions eliciting their attitude toward the then presidential candidate Ronald Reagan. Speed of response predicted the magnitude of the correlation between their attitude toward Reagan and the evaluative implications of their beliefs about his performance in the presidential debates shown on television – respondents with shorter latencies showed higher correlations between their attitudes and their beliefs about the performance of the candidate. Similar findings were reported by Houston and Fazio (1989).

Implications for interventions
The theory of spontaneous processing has some implications for interventions. For example, the model improves our understanding of problem situations in which intentions to stop health-impairing behavior patterns are likely to break down. Many health-impairing behaviors are executed automatically, except when individuals make a conscious attempt to change them. Attitudes should therefore exert a strong influence on these behavior patterns. Thus, a person keenly interested in food (i.e. an individual for whom food items typically activate a positive attitude with clear behavioral implications) may be inclined to act on that attitude unless his or her diet intentions were cognitively contrasted with this original impulse. However, such cognitive contrasting often requires effortful processing. Thus under conditions where a person's capacity or motivation for processing are low because of stress or alcohol consumption, the original intention may prevail and result in a violation of the diet intention (Ford and Kruglanski, in press). Diet programs might

therefore be improved by instructing individuals in stress management and by advising them to avoid alcohol while on a diet.

Conclusions

The theory of spontaneous processing is much less developed than the models of reasoned and planned action. In fact, only the processes mediating activation of attitudes are described in detail. The model becomes less and less definite as it progresses from attitude activation toward behavior. Furthermore, it seems plausible that the processes described by the spontaneous processing model occur prior to the activation of an attitude toward a given behavior. Thus, in the presence of stimuli relating to the attitude object, the attitude toward the object is likely to be accessed before the attitude toward some potential behavior. Thus, the spontaneous processing model should be considered supplementary rather than alternative to the models of reasoned and planned action (Eagly and Chaiken 1993).

Summary and conclusions

The first part of this chapter discussed the conditions under which attitudes are related to behavior and stressed the need for measures of attitude and behavior which are both reliable and compatible. The second part of the chapter discussed models of behavior from health and social psychology. The health belief model and protection motivation theory identified five determinants of health behavior. According to these theories, individuals are likely to engage in health protective behavior if (1) they perceive a health threat, (2) which appears serious, and (3) if they feel able to perform some action that (4) is likely to alleviate the health threat and that (5) is not too effortful or costly. The theory of reasoned action assumes that the performance or non-performance of a given behavior depends on one's intention to perform the behavior. Behavioral intentions are in turn determined by one's attitude towards performing the behavior and by subjective norms. Thus, the belief that physical exercise will lead to a number of consequences which are positively valued (attitude) and that friends, family members and/or one's partner would prefer one to lose weight (subjective norms) is likely to result in the intention to lose weight.

All of these models are theories of motivation that describe the factors influencing the formation of behavioral intentions. However, even though intentions are important determinants of behavior, actual performance depends also on other factors, such as ability, skills, information, opportunity and factors which are collectively referred to as "will-power" (i.e. the ability to maintain one's motivation during the execution of an intention). The concept of perceived control is used as a summary index of all internal and external factors that might thwart our intentions. According to the model of planned behavior, our intention to lose weight will be a function of perceived control over weight loss as well as of our attitude toward losing weight and our beliefs about the shape important others want us to have. Perceived lack of control with regard to weight loss could be due to perceived low self-efficacy (e.g. "I will never be able to control myself"), low outcome expectancy (e.g. "Even if I eat less, I will never lose any weight") and external influences (e.g. "How can I lose weight when I have to attend several business lunches every week?).

Finally, by describing the processes through which attitudes that are automatically activated may influence behavior, the spontaneous processing model developed by Fazio and colleagues improves our understanding of some of the factors that lower people's control over their actions. Thus, there is some support for the proposition that spontaneous influences of attitudes on actions are most likely to occur if our attitudes are highly accessible and if we are unmotivated or unable to deliberate about behavioral alternatives.

It is uneconomical to entertain specific theories of health behavior, such as the health belief model or protection motivation theory, unless the predictive success of these specific models is greater than that of general models, such as the theory of planned behavior. It is also unlikely that these specific models will do better in predicting behavior than the theory of planned behavior, because all of the components of the specific model can be integrated into the more general theory of planned behavior. Thus, an individual's attitude toward continuing to smoke will be the sum of the products of the positive (e.g. weight control, pleasure) and negative consequences of smoking, each weighted by its valence. Individual perceptions of susceptibility to lung cancer as well as the severity of lung cancer would therefore enter into this attitude. The attitude toward stopping, on the other hand, would reflect the perceived costs of stopping as well as beliefs about the efficacy of smoking cessation in preventing lung cancer. The concept of perceived control, as one of three determinants of intention in the theory of planned behavior, incorporates perceived self-efficacy as well as outcome expectancies. Finally, the model also considers subjective norms which have no place in the health belief model but might be important determinants of health behavior such as smoking or weight loss.

Suggestions for further reading

Ajzen, I. (1988). *Attitudes, Personality and Behavior*. Milton Keynes: Open University Press. A very readable account of the conditions under which attitudes (and personality traits) predict behavior. Discusses the principles of aggregation and compatibility as well as the theories of reasoned action and planned behavior.

Eagly, A.H. and Chaiken, S. (1993). *The Psychology of Attitudes*. Fort Worth, TX: Harcourt Brace Jovanovich. At present the most comprehensive and authoritative review of the social psychology of attitudes. Chapters 1 (nature of attitudes) and 4 (the impact of attitudes on behaviors) are most relevant to the material discussed in this chapter.

Fazio, R.H. (1990). Multiple processes by which attitudes guide behavior: The MODE model as an integrative framework. In M.P. Zanna (Ed.), *Advances in Experimental Social Psychology* (Vol. 23: 75–109). San Diego: Academic Press. Recent summary of research on the spontaneous processing model developed by Fazio and his colleagues.

Janz, N.K., and Becker, M.H. (1984). The health belief model: A decade later. *Health Education Quarterly*, II, 1–47. Description of the health belief model and review of much of the research conducted to test this model.

3 / BEYOND PERSUASION: THE MODIFICATION OF HEALTH BEHAVIOR

If we accept estimates like those from the Centers for Disease Control (1980), which suggest that a sizeable proportion of the mortality from the 10 leading causes of death in the USA is due to modifiable lifestyle factors, health psychology offers challenging opportunities to social psychologists. During the last decade, there has been a great deal of progress in social psychological understanding of processes of persuasion and attitude change (for reviews, see Petty and Cacioppo 1986; Eagly and Chaiken 1993) and health psychology would constitute a worthwhile field of application of this knowledge. Social psychologists should help to design effective mass media campaigns to inform people of the health hazards involved in smoking, drinking too much alcohol, eating food high in cholesterol, failing to exercise and other behaviors that are detrimental to their health, and to persuade them to change their lifestyles.

However, persuasion is often not enough to achieve lasting changes in health patterns. For example, even though the first report in which the US Surgeon General pointed out the health hazards of smoking had a considerable impact on smoking behavior, particularly among males, many of the people who still smoke would like to give it up but do not succeed in doing so (Leventhal and Cleary 1980). Survey data show that about one-third of all current smokers try to stop at least once per year and that only one-fifth of these succeed in any single attempt (Marlatt *et al.* 1988). Although there is probably no harm in reminding these smokers of the damage they are continuing to do to themselves, what most of them need is help not only in quitting but also in staying off cigarettes.

There are basically two stages in the modification of health behavior. The first involves the formation of an *intention to change*. Individuals have to be informed of the health hazards of certain health behaviors and to be persuaded to change. This can be achieved by public health interventions that use mass communications or other social psychological procedures of social influence. However, even if people accept a health recommendation and form the firm intention to change, they are likely to experience difficulty in *acting on these intentions* over any length of time. Thus, a second stage involves teaching people how to change and how to maintain this change. Whereas the first stage of this process can be most effectively achieved through mass media campaigns and other public health programs, with behavior such as substance abuse or excessive eating, clinical intervention may be needed at the second stage. This chapter gives a general overview of both the public health approach and the major methods of clinical intervention. The application of these methods to the modification of specific health behaviors will be described in Chapters 4 and 5.

The public health model: Motivating change

The term "public health model" is used here to refer to health promotion programs that are designed to change the behavior of large groups, such as the members of an industrial organization, or the citizens of a state or country. The objective of the public health approach is primary prevention, that is, to induce people to adopt good health habits and to change bad ones. There are basically two ways to effect this change, namely through persuasion and through modification of relevant incentives.

Persuasion is used in health education and health promotion to influence individual health beliefs and behavior. People are exposed to more or less complex messages that reflect a position advocated by a source and arguments designed to support that position. The source may be a medical expert or a public health institute and the message may point out that a specific unhealthy practice such as overeating or leading a sedentary life is likely to result in a number of very unpleasant health consequences.

Modification of relevant incentives is often employed as a public health strategy to increase the effort or costs of engaging in certain unhealthy practices or to decrease the costs of healthful practices. Thus governments may introduce economic incentives and legal measures to alter the contingencies affecting individuals as they drink, smoke or engage in other health-damaging behavior. Often persuasion and incentive modification strategies are combined. Thus a public health campaign aimed at preventing alcoholism might involve mass media messages pointing out the dangers of alcoholism, worksite health promotion programs, and changes in incentives such as an increase in the tax on alcohol or a legal restriction on the sale of alcoholic beverages.

A third public health strategy relies on passive protection through the regulation of product designs or the engineering of the physical environment to make it safer. However, this strategy is of less interest in the context of a book on social psychology and health, and will therefore only be mentioned briefly.

Theories of persuasion

Before we highlight empirical research on persuasion in laboratory and field settings, we will present a brief theoretical analysis of persuasion. This should improve our understanding of the processes or variables that mediate the impact of communications on attitudes and beliefs.

A model of systematic processing in persuasion

The information-processing paradigm proposed by McGuire (e.g. 1985) provides a useful framework for analyzing the cognitive processes involved in attitude change. In this model, the persuasive impact of a message is held to be the product of five steps: (1) attention, (2) comprehension, (3) yielding, (4) retention and (5) behavior. Thus, to have any effect, a television message warning of the health risks of unsafe sexual practices will first have to attract the attention of the audience. If viewers use this opportunity of a break between programs to get a drink (failure to attend), the appeal will not result in attitude change. However, even if viewers attend to the arguments, the message may have little impact if they do not understand the arguments because they are too complex and full of medical jargon (failure to comprehend) or if they are unwilling to accept the communicator's conclusions (failure to yield).

According to this model, the receiver must proceed through each of these steps if the communication is to have the ultimate persuasive impact. The probability of each successive step is proportional to the joint probability of the occurrence of all previous steps. Thus, even if the probability for an individual to pass through each of the stages outlined above would be 0.8, the joint probability of a persuasive message resulting in behavior change would only be 0.8^4 or 0.41. This may be one of the reasons why it is often difficult to induce behavior change through information campaigns.

The cognitive response model

The cognitive response model was developed because the low correlations between retention of message content and persuasion seemed to be inconsistent with the assumption made by McGuire that persuasion was mediated by reception and comprehension (see, however, Eagly and Chaiken 1993: 264ff.). The cognitive response approach stresses the mediating role of the individual thoughts or "cognitive responses" which recipients generate as they reflect upon persuasive communications (e.g. Greenwald 1968). According to this model, listening to a communication is like a mental discussion where the listener responds to the arguments presented in the communication. Cognitive responses reflect the content of this internal communication. The model assumes that these cognitive responses mediate the effect of persuasive messages on attitude change. Since cognitive responding is assumed to vary both in magnitude and favorability, persuasion should be a function of the *extent* of cognitive responding that occurs as well as its *favorability*.

The extent to which individuals engage in argument-relevant thinking is determined by their processing motivation and ability. The more motivated and/or able individuals are to think about the arguments contained in a communication, the more they will be able to engage in argument-relevant thinking. Whether increases in processing ability or motivation increase or decrease the persuasive impact of a communication will depend on the favorability of individual responses to the communication. The favorability of cognitive responses depends mainly on the quality of the arguments contained in a communication. A persuasive communication which contains many strong arguments will stimulate predominantly positive thoughts, whereas a communication containing weak arguments will elicit unfavorable cognitive responses. With strong arguments stimulating favorable thoughts, increases in processing motivation and/or ability should result in increased persuasion. With weak arguments eliciting unfavorable thoughts, increased motivation or ability to engage in argument-relevant thinking will decrease the persuasive impact of the communication.

These predictions have been tested in numerous experiments (see Eagly and Chaiken 1993). The impact of processing motivation on persuasion has typically been studied by manipulating the personal relevance of the topic of the communication. Consistent with predictions, increasing the personal relevance of a communication resulted in decreased persuasion for communications containing mainly weak arguments, but increased persuasion for messages which consisted of strong arguments. (Chaiken 1980; Petty *et al.* 1981).

The impact of processing ability has often been studied through the use of distraction. Distracting individuals while they are listening to a message should decrease their ability to process the message. Petty *et al.* (1976) manipulated distraction by having subjects record visual stimuli while listening to a message. The degree of distraction was varied by the frequency with which the stimuli flashed on a screen. The favorability of subjects' cognitive responses was manipulated by using either very strong or very weak arguments. In line with expectations from cognitive response theory, distraction increased persuasion for weak messages and decreased persuasion for strong messages. Furthermore, an analysis of the thoughts which subjects reported to have had during the communication, indicated that distraction inhibited the number of counterarguments for the message which contained weak arguments and reduced the number of favorable thoughts for the version consisting of strong arguments.

Dual-process models of persuasion
The two models discussed so far share the assumption that individuals who listen to a communication systematically evaluate the arguments contained in the communication to arrive at a decision about the validity of any conclusions or recommendations given. However, individuals sometimes may not be motivated or able to evaluate an argumentation and still be wanting to form an opinion on the validity of a recommended action. The dual-process models of persuasion which have recently dominated persuasion research,

namely the Elaboration Likelihood Model (e.g. Petty and Cacioppo 1986) and the Heuristic-Systematic Model (e.g. Chaiken 1980), suggest that the kind of *systematic processing* implied by the cognitive response model is only one of two different modes of information processing that mediate persuasion. If individuals are either unwilling or unable to engage in this extensive and effortful process of assessing arguments, they might base their decision to accept or reject the message on some peripheral aspect such as the credibility of the source, the length of the message or other non-content cues. This has been called *heuristic processing* (Chaiken 1980; Eagly and Chaiken 1993).

In heuristic processing, people often use simple schemas or decision rules to assess the validity of an argument. For example, people may have learned from previous experience that health recommendations from physicians tend to be more veridical than those from lay persons. They may therefore apply the rule "doctors can be trusted with regard to health issues" in response to indications that the communicator is a medical doctor, and agree with a health message. Because the individual agrees with a message without extensive thinking about the content of the arguments, dual-process theories assume that attitudes formed or changed on the basis of heuristic processing will be less stable, less resistant to counterarguments, and less predictive of subsequent behavior than those based on systematic processing.

A central prediction of dual-process models is that heuristic cues have a greater impact on attitudes than argument quality when motivation or ability to engage in issue-relevant thinking is low, whereas argument quality has a greater impact when motivation or ability to process is high. Experiments manipulating variables which were assumed to affect processing motivation or ability, such as personal relevance, time pressure, message comprehensibility or prior knowledge, have also yielded results supportive of the theory. As one would expect, the influence of peripheral cues on attitudes is low when processing ability is high, but increases substantially when recipients lack the ability to process the message extensively (e.g. Petty *et al.* 1981; Wood and Kallgren 1988).

The impact of persuasion

The major difficulty in persuading people to engage in healthful behavior patterns is that they involve immediate effort or renunciation of gratification in the here and now in order to achieve greater rewards or to avoid worse punishment in the remote future. As religious leaders discovered centuries ago, when facing similar (or even worse) problems, fear appeals can be an effective way of achieving compliance. Today, fear or threat appeals are the mainstay of most mass media health promotion campaigns. These appeals frequently consist of information that is fear-arousing and information that provokes a sense of personal vulnerability to the illness threat. They are usually followed by some recommendation that, if accepted, would reduce or avoid the danger. The effectiveness of fear appeals has been studied extensively in laboratory experiments (for reviews, see Sutton 1982; Boster and Mongeau 1984).

Persuasion in the laboratory
In a typical early study of the impact of fear appeals, smokers would be exposed to factual information about the danger of smoking in a low-threat condition. In a high-threat condition, they would in addition be exposed to a film which would make the nature of lung cancer more vivid by including a section on a lung cancer operation, showing the initial incision, the forcing apart of the ribs, and the removal of the black and diseased lung. Under both conditions, a recommendation would be given that these consequences could be avoided if subjects gave up smoking.

The vast majority of experiments on the impact of fear or threat appeals have found that higher levels of threat lead to greater persuasion than lower levels (Sutton 1982; Boster and Mongeau 1984). This effect holds for behavioral intentions as well as actual behavior, but tends to be stronger for intentions. The willingness of recipients to accept a recommendation has also been found to be affected by their perception of the effectiveness of the recommended action in averting a threat. After all, it makes little sense to spend energy and effort on some remedial action, if it is rather unlikely that such action will avert the harm. Main effects of perceived effectiveness on intentions to adopt the action have been found in a number of studies (e.g. Chu 1966; Rogers 1985).

Because interest in fear appeals eclipsed before the rise of dual-process theories, these theories have rarely been applied to this issue. From a dual-process perspective, one would predict that mild to moderate threats should increase the motivation of people who perceive themselves as vulnerable to scrutinize the message and thus result in more systematic processing. This would increase the persuasive impact of a communication for strong argumentations but decrease it for weak ones. With a higher level of fear, the emotional tension would probably disrupt people's capacity for systematic processing. This last hypothesis was supported in a persuasion experiment by Jepson and Chaiken (1990).

To conclude, the majority of studies on fear appeals have found that higher levels of threat resulted in greater persuasion than lower levels. This suggests that health messages should describe the damage likely to result from some health-impairing behavior quite vividly. However, it may be counterproductive to try to induce very high levels of fear by showing gory details of accidents to make people use seat belts or lung cancer operations in an effort to induce smokers to quit. This may not only disrupt people's capacity for systematic processing, but also motivate them to stop attending to the message. After all, subjects in the experiments on fear appeals were captive audiences and thus prevented from leaving the room or switching off their television sets, which would probably have been their normal reaction to some of the high-threat films. Health messages should further emphasize that the recommended action is effective in substantially reducing or preventing the danger and that the costs of taking that action (e.g. time, pain, money) are not out of proportion with its protective effect.

Persuasion in the field

Although laboratory studies can tell us a great deal about how to develop persuasive appeals that have maximum impact on individuals who are exposed to them, they provide only limited information about the effectiveness of persuasion in a mass media context. In real life, audiences can actively or passively avoid exposure to health messages.

There can be little doubt, however, that an extensive national campaign can produce meaningful behavioral changes in attitudes and behavior. The data on changes in per capita cigarette consumption in the USA during the latter half of this century certainly suggest that the anti-smoking campaign, which began with the first Report of the Surgeon General on Smoking and Health in 1964, had a great impact (Figure 3.1). Yet, even with such apparently clear-cut data, it is difficult to decide how much of the decline in smoking behavior should be attributed to the media

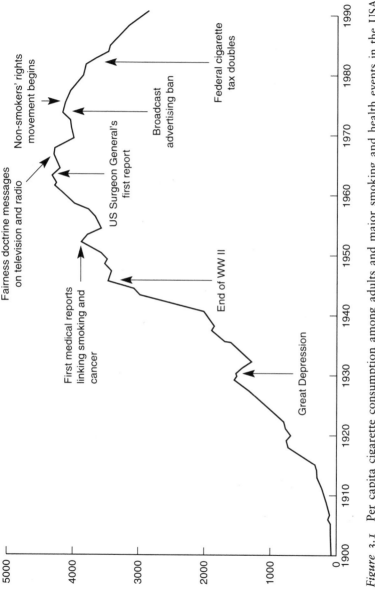

Figure 3.1 Per capita cigarette consumption among adults and major smoking and health events in the USA, 1900–1984

Source: Novotny *et al.* (1992)

campaign, and how much to other causes. For example, as a result of the changing attitude toward smoking, there were large increases in local excise taxes on cigarettes between 1964 and 1978. The increased cost of cigarettes is likely to have contributed to the decrease in cigarette consumption. Therefore, to assess the impact of the media campaign on smoking behavior, one would need a control group that is comparable in every respect to the US population but was not exposed to the campaign. Without such a comparison, we will never be certain whether smoking behavior would not have changed even without the anti-smoking campaign.

The evidence from controlled studies suggests that mass media communications usually result only in modest attitude change and even more modest behavior change (for a review, see McGuire 1985). For example, mass media campaigns persuading individuals to wear seatbelts have been rather ineffective (Robertson et al. 1974; Fhanér and Hane 1979). Similarly, a mass media campaign to encourage family planning had no effect on relevant indicators such as the sale of contraceptives, the number of unwanted pregnancies and the birthrate (Udry et al. 1972). Finally, there is no firm evidence that public education programs aimed at lowering alcohol consumption resulted in behavior change leading to a reduction in per capita consumption (for a review, see Ashley and Rankin 1988).

Limits to persuasion

Why is it so difficult to persuade people to change poor health habits, even if they accept the deleterious consequences of their behavior? One major reason is that individuals often find it very difficult to change health-impairing behavior even if they are aware of damaging their health. Thus, relapse rates are high even with clinical interventions.

A second reason is that the persuasive appeals used in studies of mass communication have frequently been developed without the benefit of social psychological theorizing. According to dual-process models, attitudes formed or changed on the basis of issue-relevant thinking are more stable, more resistant to counterarguments and more predictive of subsequent behavior than those based on heuristic processing. Therefore, if one wants to achieve stable and persistent change in health attitudes, one should design communications in a way which motivates individuals to engage in issue-relevant thinking. One also has to make sure that the arguments contained in the communication are not too complex for the intended target population. Most importantly, however, one has to develop persuasive arguments of high quality, because increases in processing motivation will only lead to increased attitude change, if the arguments contained in the communication stimulate predominantly positive responses. However, even if a communication (a) contains arguments of high quality which are (b) suited to the ability level of the audience and (c) succeed in motivating issue-related thinking, it will have little impact on the target behavior, unless it also conforms to the principle of compatibility. According to this principle, a persuasive appeal should only be effective in changing a given behavior if it addresses behavioral, normative and control beliefs which are compatible with the target behavior.

It would seem easy to fulfill those criteria. After all, most people place great value on their health. Therefore, individuals should be highly motivated to process communications which give advice on healthful behaviors. Furthermore, with all the benefits of epidemiological research on the negative impact of health-impairing behavior patterns, it should be easy to find strong arguments which have high persuasive impact.

This assessment is overly optimistic for a number of reasons. First, not everybody is interested in health issues. For example, adolescents are often not very concerned about their health and are therefore not motivated to attend to health communications (Thompson 1978). This is unfortunate, because adolescence is the time of life where many of the unhealthy practices such as smoking, drinking too much alcohol or eating the wrong diet are adopted. Once people have developed health-impairing behavior patterns, they often find it difficult to change. Second, there is some suggestion that health communications are less effective for individuals of lower socioeconomic status (Kittel *et al.* 1993). An analysis of 20 years of Belgian studies of the impact of health communications indicated that these programs were most effective for individuals of high socioeconomic status. In fact, these data suggested that 20 years of health education have resulted in an increase in the health differential which already existed between the well-off and the poor. One potential explanation for this difference could be that most of these health communications have been designed by the well educated for the well educated. Thus, less educated audiences might have been unable to understand the argumentation. Third, there is evidence that health education programs frequently violate the compatibility principle. For example, Abraham and colleagues (1992) concluded from their study of Scottish teenagers, that since young people's intentions to use condoms appear to be mainly affected by perceived barriers to condom use, educational programs should focus on acceptability barriers rather than emphasizing young people's vulnerability to infection, the severity of infection and condom effectiveness. Consistent with these conclusions, the AIDS education program developed by the Dutch Educational Television Service discussed earlier (see p. 37) failed to change intentions to use condoms, even though it was successful in affecting risk perception.

One final reason for the failure of many public health campaigns to persuade people to adopt healthful lifestyles could be due to a discrepancy between individual and population perspectives of health risks (Jeffery 1989). Public health policies are guided by the *population attributable risk*, that is, the number of excess cases of disease in a population that can be attributed to a given risk factor. Individual decision making, on the other hand, is determined by individual rather than population gain. Highest personal gain, however, is achieved when absolute risk to the individual and relative risk are both high. The problem with many health-impairing behavior patterns is that the *relative risk* – that is, the ratio of the probability of contracting the disease by individuals who engage in a risky behavior versus those who do not – is rather low. For example, a sedentary lifestyle is related to heart disease, but the relative risk is modest. And yet, because heart disease is the most common cause of death in most countries and because a sedentary lifestyle is very common, the excess burden in the population attributable to this risk factor is high.

But even if the relative risk is high, as with smoking, the absolute risk may still be so low as to make it not seem worthwhile for the individual to change. For example, even though a smoker runs a much higher risk of developing lung cancer than a non-smoker, the 10-year absolute risk of lung cancer for a 35-year-old man who is a heavy smoker is only about 0.3 per cent, and the risk of heart disease is only 0.9 per cent (Jeffery 1989). And yet, these small numbers have a tremendous significance from a population perspective. In a group of one million heavy smokers aged 35, nearly 10,000 will die (prematurely) before age 45 because of the smoking habit. From the perspective of the individual, however, the odds are heavily in favor of individual survival with or without behavior change.

Even if mass media campaigns avoid disclosing the real risks and often induce people to believe that the risks are much greater, this is probably more than compensated by the fact that people's perceptions are often distorted by a false optimism bias (Weinstein 1987). For example, since most people believe that they are far better drivers than the majority of road users, it is difficult to persuade them to exercise care and use their seatbelts.

Beyond persuasion: Changing the incentive structure

To some extent, these barriers to change can be circumvented by combining persuasion with strategies which change the rewards and costs associated with a given behavior. And in view of the uncertain effects of health promotion via mass media persuasion, it is hardly surprising that governments often decide to influence behavior by changing the rewards and costs associated with alternative courses of action rather than relying on persuasion. Thus, government policies can be introduced that alter the set of contingencies affecting individuals as they engage in health-damaging behavior (Moore and Gerstein 1981). For example, governments can increase the costs of smoking or drinking by increasing the tax on tobacco and alcohol products, they can institute stricter age limits or reduce availability by limiting sales.

Legal age restrictions

In most countries, a large segment of the population (as defined by a minimal drinking or driving age) is not permitted to buy alcohol or drive a car. Although the value of such age limits in reducing drinking problems or accident rates among the young has been doubted, the evidence from studies of changes in age limits suggests that the limits do exercise a restraining effect. For example, evaluations of the impact of changes in the minimal drinking age on alcohol and alcohol-related problems in the relevant age groups have indicated that raising the drinking age reduces both alcohol consumption and motor vehicle accidents (e.g. Ashley and Rankin 1988).

Price and taxation

One of the basic assumptions of economic theory states that, everything else being equal, the demand for a good will decrease when the price of that good is increased. The relation between changing prices and changing consumption can be expressed by price elasticities. Price elasticity reflects the way in which consumption responds to changes in price. It is defined as the percentage change in the quantity of a good demanded divided by the percentage change in the price associated with the change in demand. Thus, an elasticity of −0.7 means that a 10 per cent increase (decrease) in price would reduce (increase) the quantity of the good demanded by 7 per cent. A commodity is said to have price elasticity if the demand reacts to changes in price – that is, if the demand goes up when prices go down, or goes down when prices go up (Bruun *et al.* 1975). Similarly, income elasticity reflects the way the demand of a commodity reacts to changes in income.

There is ample evidence to demonstrate that the demand for alcoholic beverages, like the demand for most other commodities, responds to changes in price and income. In a review of econometric studies that estimated the values of price and income elasticities of alcoholic beverages for Australia, Canada, Finland, Ireland, Sweden, Great Britain and the USA, Bruun *et al.* (1975) concluded that, everything else remaining equal, a rise in alcohol prices had generally led to a drop in the consumption of alcohol, whereas an increase in the income of consumers generally led to a rise in alcohol consumption. There is similar evidence for smoking, although less research seems to have been conducted on this issue (for reviews, see Warner 1981, 1986; Walsh and Gordon 1986).

Summary and conclusions

If one compares the effectiveness of public health strategies that use persuasion and those that change the contingencies associated with a given behavior (e.g. price), the latter strategy may seem more effective. However, there are limitations to the use of monetary incentives or legal sanctions to influence health behavior which do not apply to persuasion. First, these strategies cannot be applied to all health behaviors. Whereas it is widely accepted that governments should control the price of tobacco products and alcohol, a law forcing people to jog daily would be unacceptable and difficult to enforce. Second, the use of monetary incentives or legal sanctions to control behavior might weaken internal control mechanisms that may have existed beforehand. Research on the effects of extrinsic incentives on intrinsic motivation and performance has demonstrated that performance of an intrinsically enjoyable task will decrease once people are given some reward for performing that task (e.g. Lepper and Greene 1978). For example, if health insurance companies decided to offer lower rates to people who engage in regular physical exercise, such financial incentives might undermine the intrinsic motivation of people who exercise because they enjoy doing this.

Mass media communications can alert people to health risks that they might not otherwise learn about (Taylor 1991). Thus, public health education through the mass media has already resulted in a major change in health attitudes, which in turn may have increased popular acceptance of legal actions curbing health-impairing behavior. For example, Warner (1981) attributed the large growth in state and local excise taxes for cigarettes between 1964 and 1972 to the anti-smoking campaign. The anti-smoking campaign in the USA is also an illustration of the fact that persuasion and incentive-related strategies do not exclude each other and are probably most effective when used in combination. Thus, the anti-smoking campaign resulted in a non-smoking ethos which was probably responsible for the legislative successes of the non-smokers' rights movements during the 1970s and 1980s.

Settings for health promotion

Following our review of public health approaches to health promotion, this section gives a few examples of the settings in which these strategies have been applied. We will begin this discussion with a somewhat unusual setting for a *public* health measure, namely the physician's office.

The physician's office

Although prevention has not been a strong component of traditional medical practice, medical school curricula are increasingly emphasizing the value of diagnosing health-impairing habits in healthy people and of advising them to change (Taylor 1991). As health experts who usually have a relationship of trust with their patients, physicians are particularly credible agents for inducing changes in health behavior. Health advice is therefore more likely to be followed if it is issued by one's personal physician rather than some anonymous mass media source. Thus, physicians can become influential in health promotion, by merely advising patients to change health-impairing behavior. For example, there is empirical evidence to demonstrate that advice given to patients to stop smoking resulted in a moderate though significant reduction in the number of people who smoked (e.g. Russell *et al.* 1979).

Physicians are likely to be even more effective in their traditional role of giving health recommendations if they act on the basis of medical tests and examinations. For example, the advice to eat a low cholesterol diet is more likely to be followed by a patient who has just received feedback that his or her serum cholesterol values are high, than without such feedback. To increase adherence in these situations, however, it is important that the information is made understandable to the patient and that specific recommendations are given. Instead of merely telling patients that they should lower their cholesterol intake, specific goals should be set (Locke and Latham 1990). Furthermore, the physician (or a dietitian working with the physician) should give specific information on the cholesterol content of various foods to help patients reach these goals. Finally, doctors and patients should agree on a date for new tests to be conducted to allow feedback on the success of these measures.

Schools

The school system is an ideal place for health promotion because, potentially, one can reach the total population and reach them early enough to prevent health-impairing habits from developing. For example, schools have been particularly active in instituting anti-smoking programs (for reviews, see Leventhal and Cleary 1980; Flay 1985; Best *et al.* 1988; Cleary *et al.* 1988). These programs vary from lectures by school principals or physicians to fear-arousing films, teacher participation (e.g. introducing material on smoking into science and hygiene classes) and student participation (e.g.

anti-smoking essays, group discussions). Evaluations of these programs suggest that so far only moderate reductions in the number of students who start smoking have been achieved (Flay 1985). The reason may be that these programs were mainly designed to prevent initial attempts at smoking. They are not very successful in preventing adolescents who have already experimented with cigarettes from turning into regular smokers. These problems may be overcome by new programs which incorporate measures aimed at slowing or reversing the progression from experimental to regular smoker (e.g. Leventhal et al. 1988).

Worksite

The worksite is an advantageous setting for conducting health promotion activities because a very large number of people can be reached on a regular basis. This allows the use of strategies that combine the public health approach with some of the clinical approaches to be discussed later. There is also a potential for manipulation of the social and physical environments in order to create positive incentives for healthful behavior. Furthermore, the possibility of reduced health care costs and absenteeism make such interventions attractive for organizations (Cataldo and Coates 1986; Terborg 1988). The advantages of instituting such worksite health promotion programs seem to have been recognized by many industrial organizations. Thus, a recently conducted US national survey of worksite health promotion programs based on a random sample of worksites with 50 or more employees, found that 65.5 per cent of these worksites reported at least one health promotion activity (Fielding and Piserchia 1989).

Taylor (1991) discussed three ways in which companies have dealt with the poor health habits of their employees. The first is through on-the-job programs that help employees to practice better health behavior. Thus, the most commonly offered health promotion activities consist of advice on exercise, stress management, smoking cessation, weight loss, nutrition and hypertension detection and control (Fielding 1986; Terborg 1988). A second way in which industry has promoted good health habits is by structuring the working environment in ways that help employees to engage in healthy activities. For example, companies might provide on-site health clubs, or open restaurants that provide a balanced diet, low in fat, sugar and cholesterol. Very few industries use the third approach, namely offering monetary incentives for healthy behavior (Terborg 1988). Although there is great enthusiasm about the efficacy of these programs, there has been only limited evaluative research to support these convictions (Fielding 1986, 1991; Terborg 1988). However, some of the programs that have been evaluated, such as Johnson and Johnson's "Live for Life" or Control Data's "Staywell", have been quite effective (Fielding 1991; Jose and Anderson 1991).

Community

This type of intervention incorporates a variety of different approaches, ranging from door-to-door or mass media information campaigns telling people about the availability of a breast cancer screening program to a diet modification program that recruits through community institutions. Evaluation of community-based interventions using quasi-experimental control group designs suggest that these interventions can be quite effective (e.g. Farquhar et al. 1977; Egger et al. 1983; Puska et al. 1985).

One of the best-known community programs aimed at changing behavioral risk factors for cardiovascular diseases – the Stanford-Three-Community Study – exposed several communities to a mass-media campaign concerning smoking, diet and exercise via television, radio, newspapers, posters and printed materials sent by mail. In one of the communities, the media campaign was even supplemented by face-to-face counselling for a small subset of high-risk individuals. A control community was not exposed to the campaign. The media campaign increased people's knowledge about cardiac risk and resulted in modest improvements in dietary preferences and other cardiac risk factors (Farquhar et al. 1977; Meyer et al. 1980).

The North Karelia Project, a large-scale community intervention conducted in northern Finland, resulted in a more substantial reduction in coronary risk factors (Puska et al. 1985). An intensive educational campaign was implemented using the news services, physicians and public health nurses who staffed community health centers. An assessment of the effectiveness of these programs based on self-report data showed that, compared to a neighboring province used as a control group and not exposed to the campaign, there was a considerable improvement in several dietary habits in North Karelia (especially concerning fat intake). There was also a net reduction in smoking, as well as small but significant net reductions in serum cholesterol levels and blood pressure. Most importantly, however, there was a 24 per cent decline in cardiovascular death in North Karelia, compared with a 12 per cent decline nationwide in Finland. Although the fact that the project was instituted in response to concerns among the North Karelia population about the extremely high heart disease rate in the area limits the generalizability of these results, findings such as these suggest that community-based interventions can be effective in changing health-impairing behavior patterns.

Summary and conclusions

Drawing on different settings for health promotion allows one to reach different sections of the population. Therefore, there are good reasons for pursuing each of the venues of health habit change. Community interventions and school programs can be used to educate the population about unhealthy lifestyles and to motivate people either not to adopt health-impairing behaviors or to change such behaviors if they have already been adopted. Physicians can also be an important part of this endeavor. Schools are potentially able to play an important role in persuading individuals not to adopt certain unhealthy behaviors such as smoking, drug use and excessive drinking. Industrial organizations, on the other hand, can become important sources of motivation for individuals to change health-impairing habits. Because large industrial organizations can often also afford to employ professional counsellors in their health promotion classes, they can effectively combine the public health and clinical therapy approaches.

The therapy model: Changing and maintaining change

Most people who seek therapy for problematic health behavior will first have attempted to achieve the desired change on their own (Schachter 1982). Thus 90 per cent of an estimated 37 million people who stopped smoking in the two decades following the US Surgeon General's first report linking smoking to cancer have done so unaided (American Cancer Society 1986). After all, therapy is expensive and most people believe that they are quite capable of giving up smoking or losing weight on their own, at least until they try to do so.

Unlike the public health model, most therapy programs involve a one-to-one relationship where "patients" and therapists are in dyadic interaction, although group treatments and self-therapy programs are also used (Leventhal and Cleary 1980). Because people who come to therapy programs have already decided to change and are motivated to act on their decision, the function of therapy programs is not to *persuade* people to change but to help them to *achieve* and maintain the desired change.

Cognitive-behavioral treatment procedures

Most therapy directed at changing problematic health behavior has relied on behavioral techniques, although cognitive components have been included in more recent behavioral treatment programs. Behavioral treatment procedures can be distinguished from other therapeutic orientations in that they involve one or a number of specific techniques that use learning-based principles to change behavior. More recently, therapeutic methods designed to impact specifically on cognitive variables have become standard components of every contemporary approach to behavioral treatment (Ingram and Scott 1990).

The major behavioral or cognitive techniques that have been used in therapies aimed at changing health-impairing behavior patterns are classical or Pavlovian conditioning (e.g. aversion therapies), operant procedures (e.g. contingency management, contingency contracting), self-management procedures, skill training and cognitive restructuring. Earlier therapies often relied on only one of these techniques (narrow band approach). Present-day behavioral clinicians generally use a multitude of different techniques within one treatment program. The obvious drawback of such a "broadspectrum behavioral approach" is that it is difficult to know at the end of a successful therapy, which aspect or aspects of the treatment package were really effective.

This section outlines the theoretical principles underlying these therapeutic procedures. A more detailed description of specific therapies (e.g. for alcoholism, obesity and smoking), as well as an evaluation of their effectiveness, will be given in Chapter 4.

Classical conditioning

Classical conditioning was first described in 1927 by the Russian physiologist Pavlov, who in research on the digestive system of dogs, observed that many of these animals already began to salivate when they heard the footsteps of the assistant who normally fed them. Pavlov reasoned that the normal response to food (salivating) had become linked to the assistant's footsteps. Thus, by regularly preceding the stimulus that normally elicits salivation (i.e. the food), the assistant's footsteps had gained the power to elicit this response. Expressed more technically, salivation had become conditioned to the sound of the steps. Salivation in response to food (the unconditioned stimulus for this type of response) would be called an *unconditioned* response; salivation elicited by the sound of footsteps (the conditioned stimulus) would be called a *conditioned* response.

The first study which demonstrated that classical conditioning can be used to condition aversive reactions in humans was an experiment by Watson and Raynor (1920), in which they used a loud noise to instill fear of laboratory rats in a little boy. The noise was a very loud bang that was known to make the child cry and to display all signs of fear. Watson and Raynor demonstrated that the fear reaction which had initially been elicited by the noise became conditioned to the rat. Following this principle, Watson and Raynor (1920) developed the model for aversion therapy.

Early attempts at aversion therapy relied on electric shock (e.g. McGuire and Vallance 1964). However, although shocks are quite effective with laboratory animals, they did not seem to work well with humans. Modern behavior therapies therefore employ aversive reactions that are *relevant* to the response that needs to be changed. Thus, aversion therapy with alcoholics has used vomiting-inducing drugs. The alcoholic is then given alcohol just a few minutes before nausea and vomiting occurs (e.g. Lemers and Voegtlin 1950). Similarly, smokers might be induced to smoke continually, inhaling every 6–8 seconds until they cannot stand it any longer (Lichtenstein and Danaher 1975). Sometimes aversion therapy uses imaginary rather than real stimuli to arouse aversion (e.g. Elkins 1980). In this procedure, both the target behavior and the aversive stimulus are presented through imagination. For example, the subject has first to imagine him or herself preparing to smoke and then experiencing nausea and vomiting.

Operant conditioning

Operant procedures modify behavior by manipulating the consequences of such behavior. They involve the contingent presentation (or withdrawal) of rewards and punishments in order to increase desirable or decrease undesirable behavior. Behavioral theorists assume that health behaviors, like any other behavior, have been learned through processes of operant conditioning. For example, a widely accepted theory of alcohol abuse, the Tension Reduction Hypothesis, assumes that alcohol is consumed because it reduces tension. By lowering tension, and thus reducing an aversive drive state, alcohol consumption has reinforcing properties. Cigarette smoking may have similar tension-reducing functions.

Like the early forms of aversive conditioning, operant procedures initially used electric shocks to change behavior. Because these procedures did not prove to have lasting effects, present-day operant procedures frequently employ some form of contingency management. For example, smokers or alcoholics may agree with their therapist on some set of rewards or punishments that will be enacted, contingent on their behavior.

Self-management procedures

Classical and operant conditioning procedures are based on the assumption that the forces shaping a person's life lie primarily in the external environment. In contrast, self-management procedures are based on the assumption that individuals can organize their environment in ways which make certain behaviors more likely (e.g. Miller and Munoz 1976). For example, individuals can reward themselves for reaching certain behavioral goals (e.g. for losing a certain amount of weight) or punish themselves for transgressing a predetermined rule (i.e. not to drink before the evening).

Goal-setting may be the most effective component of self-management. The application of self-reinforcement always involves some goal that has to be reached for the reinforcement to be applied. That this is an important determinant of the effectiveness of such procedures is suggested by research on goal setting in the context of task performance in industry. This work has consistently demonstrated that setting specific and challenging goals and providing relevant feedback leads to substantial increases in performance (for a review see Locke and Latham 1990). Specific goals are likely to result in specific behavioral intentions. The greater effectiveness of specific over more global goals would therefore also be consistent with predictions derived from the models of reasoned action or planned behavior. Because self-reinforcements are usually made dependent on reaching very specific goals, and because individuals provide themselves with relevant feedback through self-monitoring, these procedures are comparable to those used in goal-setting research.

Skill training

Skill training procedures have been used both as a primary treatment strategy in narrow-band approaches and as one of a number of approaches in broad spectrum programs (Riley *et al.* 1987). The main assumption underlying skill-training techniques is that people engage in health impairing behavior because they lack certain skills. For example, people might become alcoholics because they lack the appropriate strategy to cope with stress (Riley *et al.* 1987). Relapsed addicts frequently report that stress and negative emotional states often immediately preceded their return to drug use (e.g. Baer and Lichtenstein 1988; Bliss *et al.* 1989). By providing individuals with the skills for coping with such stressful situations, there will be an alternative response to cope with the problem. This should reduce the need to turn to cigarettes or alcohol in order to be able to cope.

Cognitive restructuring

These techniques help patients to identify and correct the self-defeating thoughts which are frequently associated with emotional upset and relapse experiences. For example, Mahoney and Mahoney (1976) described the irrational and maladaptive cognitions that dieters often experience. These include thoughts about the impossibility of weight loss, the adoption of unrealistic goals which are soon disappointed, and self-disparaging statements. Using the methods of Beck (1976) and Meichenbaum (1977), patients are taught to discredit these arguments.

Relapse and relapse prevention

One distressing aspect of changing problematic health behavior either through therapy or unaided is that people are often unable to maintain their changed habits. Thus relapse rates for addictions range from 50 per cent to 90 per cent with approximately two-thirds of the relapses occurring within the first 90 days (Marlatt and Gordon, 1980; Marlatt 1985; Brownell *et al.* 1986). Similarly, in the field of weight control, few of the dieters who succeed in losing substantial amounts of weight are able to maintain their losses for any significant period of time (Sternberg, 1985).

Despite the high probability that clients who undergo therapy to change some health impairing habit will experience a relapse soon after the end of their therapy, this possibility used not to be discussed (or even acknowledged) during therapy. Thus when it happened, clients were unprepared to cope with relapse. During the last decade, this attitude has changed and specific relapse prevention approaches have been developed (e.g. Marlatt and Gordon 1985; Brownell *et al.* 1986). These models emphasize the similarities in the precipitating conditions and consequences of relapse experiences across different domains of health behavior.

The most comprehensive theory of the relapse process has been developed by Marlatt and colleagues (Marlatt and Gordon 1980; Marlatt 1985). Their cognitive behavioral model of relapse (Figure 3.2.) integrates elements from social psychological theories such as social learning, attribution, and dissonance theory to account for the relapse process.

Central to the model is the concept of *perceived control* or *self-efficacy* (Bandura 1986). It is assumed that individuals who manage to maintain abstinence or to comply with some other rule regarding the target behavior (e.g. controlled drinking, smoking reduction, dieting) experience a sense of control. This sense of control, which will become stronger the longer the period of abstinence maintenance or successful rule following, will be threatened when individuals encounter a high-risk situation. *High-risk situations* are situations which increase the risk of relapse.

Cummings and colleagues (1980) analyzed more than 300 initial relapse episodes obtained from clients with a variety of problem behaviors such as problem drinking, smoking, heroin addiction, compulsive gambling, and overeating. On the basis of these reports, three primary high-risk situations that were associated with almost three-quarters of all the relapses could be identified. Relapses happened most often in the presence of *negative emotional states* (35 per cent of all relapses) such as depression, anxiety, or stress. For example, depression resulting from the failure to pass

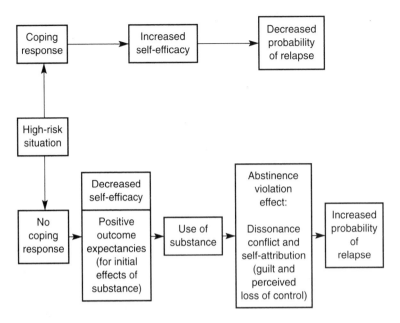

Figure 3.2   A cognitive-behavioral model of the relapse process
Source: Adapted from Marlatt (1985)

an exam would significantly increase the likelihood of relapse. *Interpersonal conflicts* (16 per cent of the relapses) also appear to be a frequent antecedent of relapse. Thus, people who have gone through the break-up of a relationship or had a conflict with a family member or their boss might take a drink or smoke a cigarette in an attempt to calm themselves. *Social pressure* (20 per cent of the relapses) is another frequent cause of relapse, involving either direct social influence from people who exert pressure on the individual to engage in the taboo behavior or indirect pressure via modelling (e.g. being in the presence of others who engage in the same target behavior).

Although Cummings and colleagues (1980) found that "urges and temptations" were associated with only 6 per cent of the relapse situations and "negative physical states" with only 7 per cent of the situations, it seems likely that physiological factors also play a major role in triggering relapse. For example, in the cases of smoking and alcoholism, such physiological influences are related to withdrawal, and may prompt some relapse, especially shortly after initial efforts to change behavior. There are conditioned associations between specific cues and physiological responses that may lead to "urges" or "cravings" to engage in the habit. Different but also influential physiological factors may be involved in obesity. Even though food does not seem to be addictive in the way that cigarettes and alcohol are, the physiological pressure to regain lost weight may be extremely powerful (Brownell *et al.* 1986). Genetic factors that are implicated in alcoholism and obesity may also operate via physiological urges (e.g. Goodwin *et al.* 1973; Stunkard *et al.* 1986).

If individuals manage to cope effectively with the high-risk situation, the probability of relapse will decrease significantly. One reason for this emphasized by Marlatt (1980), is that individuals who cope successfully will have validated their sense of control. They will therefore expect to cope with future high-risk situations. This expectancy is closely associated with the notions of self-efficacy (Bandura 1986) and perceived control (Ajzen 1988). High self-efficacy or high perceived control are positively related to behavioral intentions. Individuals are more motivated to engage in a behavior if they perceive their ability to perform that behavior successfully as high rather than low.

A somewhat different but complementary explanation could be derived from dissonance theory. Dissonance theory would suggest that the voluntary decision to refrain from performing a desirable behavior should lead to increased derogation of that behavior (c.f. Aronson and Carlsmith 1963). For example, former smokers who were tempted to smoke but refrained should be motivated to justify their behavior by further elaborating the negative consequences of smoking.

In contrast, failure to cope with the high-risk situation should decrease the sense of control or self-efficacy. The risk of failure should be particularly high if the situation also involves the temptation to engage in the prohibited behavior as a means of coping with the stress. For example, if an individual is very anxious about the outcome of some examination and also feels that smoking a cigarette or having a drink would calm him or her down, the risk of relapse is very high. Thus, the combination of being unable to cope effectively in a high risk situation, combined with the positive outcome expectancies for the effects of the old habitual coping behavior greatly increases the probability of an initial relapse.

Most people who attempt to change a health impairing habit

such as smoking or drinking perceive "stopping" in a "once and for all" manner. Thus, the transgression of an absolute rule will result in what Marlatt and Gordon (1980) termed the *abstinence violation effect* (i.e. the inference that the failure to remain abstinent is an indication of one's complete lack of will-power and self-control). However, because similar effects can be observed in dieters who have violated their diet norm, one should perhaps use the more general concept of a *goal violation effect* (Polivy and Herman 1987).

One major reason for the abstinence or goal violation effect is *self-attribution*. The concept of attribution refers to the processes by which individuals arrive at causal explanations for their own or other people's actions (Heider 1958). These explanations can vary on a continuum that ranges from attributions to internal causes to attributions to external causes. Examples of internal causes would be personality, ability or motivation. Examples of external causes would be task difficulty, or social pressure. Individuals who relapse are likely to make internal attributions. They tend to blame the relapse on personal weakness or failure and to interpret it as evidence of their lack of will-power and their inability to resist temptation. This self-attribution will further decrease the individual's sense of self-efficacy and control.

A second reason for the abstinence or goal violation effect is *dissonance*. The flagrant violation of a dietary goal or abstinence rule would also be inconsistent with the individual's self-concept (as a dieter or abstainer) and therefore arouse dissonance. Dissonance is an aversive internal state which is assumed to motivate individuals to reduce dissonance (Festinger 1957). In the case of violations of abstention rules, dissonance can either be reduced by changing one's self-image or by changing one's attitude towards abstention. Thus, ex-smokers who relapse could reduce their dissonance either by deciding that they have no will-power or by persuading themselves that smoking is not so bad after all. Obviously, both mechanisms of dissonance reduction would increase the risk of future relapse.

According to this analysis, the first step to take in the prevention of relapse is to teach clients to recognize high-risk situations that are likely to trigger a relapse (Marlatt 1985). The second step involves teaching them the coping skills that are necessary to master the high risk situation. Such relapse prevention techniques have now been tested with a variety of health behaviors including alcohol abstinence (e.g. Chaney *et al.* 1978), smoking (e.g. Shiffman *et al.* 1985), and weight control (Sternberg, 1985). Although there is evidence that such programs can produce higher rates of adherence relative to programs with no relapse prevention, it is too early to draw any firm conclusions.

Summary and conclusions

This chapter presented and discussed two types of approaches to the modification of health behavior, the public health model and the therapy model. The public health model involves health promotion programs that are designed to change the behavior of large groups (e.g. members of industrial organizations, students of a school, citizens of a community or even the population of a country). Three major strategies are used to achieve this objective: persuasive appeals, economic incentives and legal measures.

Mass media health appeals are quite effective in increasing people's knowledge of certain health hazards but they are much less effective in changing their behavior. As Jeffery (1989) has pointed out, one reason for the failure of health campaigns to induce significant behavior change is that the objectives of these campaigns are usually selected from a population, rather than an individual, perspective. Individuals are most likely to change their behavior if they can be persuaded that such a change would considerably reduce their personal risk of contracting some threatening disease.

Unfortunately, many of the risk factors that are important from a public health perspective are associated with a low or moderate personal risk. Their importance is due to the fact that they are common in a population. Jeffery (1989) suggested that under these conditions, where persuasion is unlikely to influence behavior, it may be more effective to rely on economic incentives or legal measures to induce behavior change.

As the anti-smoking campaign of the 1960s and 1970s illustrated, public health approaches can achieve significant behavior change if extensive media campaigns are combined with economic and legal measures. Thus, the mass media campaign that was initiated by the report of the US Surgeon General is likely to have played a causal role in the global change of attitudes toward smoking. This general change in climate was probably responsible for the increases in local and state taxation during the late 1960s and for the legislative successes of the non-smokers' rights movements during the 1970s.

However, the example of smoking can also serve to illustrate the weaknesses of the public health approach. It has been very successful in conveying information about the health risk of smoking – nearly everyone in the US now believes that cigarette smoking is hazardous. It has been less successful in changing behavior. Nearly one-third of the US population continues to smoke, despite the considerable reduction in the prevalence of smoking during recent decades.

The fact that many of the people who smoke today would like to stop suggests that a sizeable proportion of those individuals have been unable to stop on their own and would profit from clinical therapy. Thus, even though educational campaigns can be effective in motivating individuals to change, good intentions are often not enough in the case of health-impairing behavior such as substance abuse or excessive eating. By teaching people strategies that help them to maintain the motivation and to execute their intention to change, clinical therapy can make an important contribution to changing these sorts of behaviors.

Thus, public health strategies and clinical therapy are complementary rather than contradictory approaches. To decide to undergo therapy, individuals must first be aware of having a problem and be willing to do something about it. Although in the case of problems such as alcoholism or obesity public health education may be less instrumental in creating problem awareness, with other problems health education has certainly played an important role in creating awareness.

Suggestions for further reading

Eagly, A.H. and Chaiken, S. (1993). *The Psychology of Attitudes*. Fort Worth, TX: Harcourt Brace Jovanovich. A comprehensive and authoritative review of the social psychology of attitudes. Chapters 6 and 7 discuss the process theories of attitude formation and change.

Jeffery, R.W. (1989). Risk behaviors and health: contrasting individual and population perspectives. *American Psychologist*, 44, 1194–1202. Argues that the discrepancy between the individual and the population perspective of health risks is responsible for the failure of many public health campaigns to influence health behavior.

Marlatt, G.A. and Gordon, J.R. (Eds) (1985). *Relapse Prevention*. New York: Guilford. The book provides a comprehensive approach to relapse prevention.

Puska, P., Nissinen, A., Tuomilehto, J., Salonen, J.T., Koskela, K., McAlister, A., Kottke, T.E., Maccoby, N. and Farquhar, J.W. (1985). The community-based strategy to prevent coronary heart disease: Conclusions from ten years of the North Karelia Project. In L. Breslow, J.E. Fielding and L.B. Lave (Eds). *Annual Review of Public Health* Vol. 6, pp. 147–94). Palo Alto, CA: Annual Reviews Inc. Reviews the main findings of the North Karelia project, a large scale community intervention aimed at changing behavioral risk factors for cardiovascular disease.

Weinstein, N.D. (1987). Unrealistic optimism about susceptibility to health problems: Conclusions from a community-wide sample. *Journal of Behavioral Medicine*, 10, 481–500. Discusses the optimism bias in the perception of health risks.

4 / BEHAVIOR AND HEALTH: EXCESSIVE APPETITES

In the two previous chapters we examined determinants of health behavior and the effectiveness of strategies for change. The next two chapters will discuss the major behavioral risk factors that have been linked to health. We divide our discussion of behavior and health into two. Chapter 4 covers health-impairing behavior related to excessive appetites, such as smoking, drinking too much alcohol and overeating (Orford 1985). These are appetitive behaviors that, once excessive, are exceedingly difficult to control. People who want to change often enter counseling or therapy programs to help them to act according to their intentions.

In contrast, self-protective behaviors such as eating a healthy diet, exercising, safeguarding oneself against the risk of injury from accidents (e.g. wearing a seatbelt), and avoiding behavior associated with contracting AIDS (needle sharing, unprotected sex), which we discuss in Chapter 5, are generally somewhat more under the voluntary control of the individual.

The structure of our discussion of behavioral risk factors is similar in both chapters. Each begins with a critical review of the empirical evidence that links these behaviors to negative health consequences. It will be shown that this relationship is well established in some cases (e.g. smoking, needle sharing, promiscuous sex), but that the evidence is rather less persuasive in others (e.g. dietary cholesterol). After a discussion of theories of the development and maintenance of these behaviors, we then discuss the effectiveness of strategies of attitude and behavior change in modifying the risk of health impairment.

Smoking

Smoking and health

Cigarette smoking has been identified as the single most important source of preventable mortality and morbidity in each of the reports of the US Surgeon General since 1964 (Fielding 1985a, b). It has been estimated that an average of $5\frac{1}{2}$ minutes of life are lost for each cigarette smoked and that deaths from cigarette smoking in the USA exceed 320,000 annually (American Cancer Society 1986). This is more than the total number of American lives lost in the First World War, Korea and Vietnam combined. To claim an equivalent share of lives, the airline industry would have to experience three jumbo jet crashes every day of the year (Walsh and Gordon 1986).

Of the deaths each year due to coronary heart disease (the leading cause of death in most industrialized countries), 30–40 per cent can be attributed to cigarette smoking (Fielding 1985a, b). Overall, the mortality from heart disease in the USA is 70 per cent greater for smokers than non-smokers (US Department of Health and Human Services 1985). Similar excessive rates have been reported for Canada, the UK, Scandinavia and Japan (Pooling Project Research Group 1978).

The second leading cause of death in the USA and other affluent industrial nations is cancer, of which lung cancer is responsible for more deaths than any other cancer. In the USA, it accounts for 25 per cent of cancer mortality and 5 per cent of all deaths (Fielding 1985a). Between 80 and 85 per cent of deaths from lung cancer have been attributed to smoking (US Department of Health and Human Services 1982). However, contrary to popular beliefs, coronary heart disease and not lung cancer is the major cause of smoking-related deaths, because many more people die of heart disease than of lung cancer. In fact, lung cancer is only responsible for one-seventh of the excess mortality attributed to smoking (Krüger and Schmidt 1989).

Morbidity is also considerably higher among smokers than among non-smokers. Current smokers report more chronic bronchitis, emphysema, chronic sinusitis, peptic ulcers and arteriosclerotic heart disease than do persons who have never smoked (Schwartz 1987). Data from the National Health Interview Survey conducted in the USA in 1974 suggest that there are more than 81 million excess work days lost and more than 145 million excess days of bed disability per year because of smoking (Schwartz 1987).

The risk of morbidity and mortality for pipe and cigar smokers who do not inhale deeply is somewhat smaller than that for cigarette smokers, but still considerably higher than that for non-smokers (Fielding 1985a, b). It is less clear whether smokers of filter cigarettes run a lower risk of morbidity and mortality than smokers of non-filter cigarettes. Although there is some evidence that changing from non-filter to filter cigarettes lowers the risk of lung cancer it does not seem to reduce the risk of developing congestive heart disease (Fielding 1985a, b). Most surprisingly, a recent large-scale study conducted in Germany even found that smokers of filter cigarettes died on average 4 years earlier than smokers of non-filter cigarettes (Krüger and Schmidt 1989).

Although there can be no doubt that smoking is unhealthy, estimates of smoking-related morbidity and mortality are likely to exaggerate the direct impact of smoking on health. Such estimates are usually based on the difference between the age-adjusted morbidity and mortality rates of smokers and non-smokers. To attribute these differences to smoking would only be justified if smokers did not differ from non-smokers except with respect to their smoking.

This is clearly not the case. People who smoke live unhealthily in other respects as well, and this could contribute to their elevated mortality risk. A national survey of behavioral risk factors conducted in the USA (Remington et al. 1985) indicated that compared with non-smokers, smokers had higher age-adjusted rates of "acute drinking" (five or more alcoholic drinks per occasion at least once a month) and "chronic drinking" (averaging two or more alcoholic drinks per day), more episodes of driving while intoxicated, and lower use of seatbelts. Even ex-smokers resemble smokers more than non-smokers in their higher consumption of alcohol (Carmody et al. 1985). Finally, Castro et al. (1989) reported that compared with non-smokers, both light and moderate-to-heavy cigarette smokers exhibited less positive health attitudes. Moderate-to-heavy smokers exhibited a lower consciousness about their health and engaged more often in behaviors that increase the risk of coronary illness in addition to smoking. These unhealthy attitudes and behaviors are likely to further impair the coronary health of smokers and contribute to their higher mortality from coronary heart diseases. However, such unhealthy practices of smokers could not account for their elevated lung cancer mortality risk.

Smokers not only damage their own health, they also endanger the health of others. Epidemiological data suggest that cigarette use during pregnancy may be related to spontaneous abortion, premature birth, low birthweight, and the death of the infant during the first day of life (McGinnis *et al.* 1987; Kaplan 1988). There is also evidence from studies assessing mortality from lung cancer among non-smoking persons exposed to smoking spouses that these "involuntary" or "passive" smokers have an elevated risk of lung cancer (e.g. Trichopoulos *et al.* 1983; Garfinkel *et al.* 1985; Akiba *et al.* 1986; Humble *et al.* 1987; Pershagen *et al.* 1987; Helsing *et al.* 1988). In the USA, such findings have led to the introduction of much more stringent restrictions in the places where tobacco can be smoked (US Department of Health and Human Services 1986; Eriksen *et al.* 1988). Similar restrictions are now being considered in England after the first court case in which £15,000 in damages was awarded to an employee who claimed that sitting near seven chain-smokers for 14 months had permanently affected her health (*Independent on Sunday*, 31 January 1993). There are even reports that people who believe that their health was damaged in childhood by passive smoking have begun taking legal advice about suing their parents (*Independent on Sunday*, 31 January 1993).

Theories of smoking

In attempting to explain why people smoke, we have to distinguish between becoming a smoker and maintaining the habit. Social pressure from peers or elder siblings is probably the prime factor in experimenting with smoking (Leventhal and Cleary 1980; Spielberger 1986). This initial experimentation is a crucial step. Some data suggest that 85–90 per cent of those who smoke four cigarettes become regular smokers (Salber *et al.* 1963). This is one of the reasons why the prevention of smoking should begin in school and target young people before they have experimented with smoking (Best *et al.* 1988).

Reasons for smoking
The reasons smokers give for why they maintain the habit, once initiated, have been analyzed extensively (Ikard *et al.* 1969;

Leventhal and Avis 1976; Spielberger 1986). Factor analyses of self-report data collected from samples of smokers have led to very similar factor structures. For example, a study conducted by Leventhal and Avis (1976) resulted in the following factors: pleasure–taste (e.g. "I like the taste of tobacco"); addiction (e.g. "I get a real gnawing hunger for a cigarette when I haven't smoked for a while"); habit (e.g. "I smoke cigarettes automatically without even being aware of it"); anxiety (e.g. "When I am nervous in social situations, I smoke"); stimulation (e.g. "Smoking makes me feel more awake"); social rewards (e.g. "I smoke to be sociable"); and fiddle ("Handling a cigarette is part of the enjoyment of smoking").

Leventhal and Avis (1976) and Ikard and Tomkins (1973) examined the validity of these reports by dividing subjects on the basis of their responses to such questionnaires into high and low scorers on a particular dimension. When the actual smoking behavior of these subjects was examined under experimentally manipulated conditions, their behavior validated their reported reasons for smoking. For example, when smokers were given cigarettes adulterated with vinegar, those high on the pleasure–taste factor showed a sharp drop in the number of cigarettes smoked, but those low on the factor did not (Leventhal and Avis 1976). When asked to monitor their smoking by filling out a card for each cigarette smoked, habit smokers significantly reduced their smoking, whereas pleasure–taste smokers did not (Leventhal and Avis 1976). Finally, there was more smoking during and after a fear-arousing film by smokers who used smoking for anxiety reduction (Ikard and Tomkins 1973). Both studies also found that addicts suffered the most during periods of deprivation. These findings suggest that the functions of smoking are reliably reported and that some of these self-reports identify the conditions that stimulate smoking (Leventhal and Cleary 1980). This is obviously an important finding for the development of intervention strategies.

Psychological theories
Research on reasons for smoking was originally stimulated by Tomkins' (1966) affect–control model. Like many before him, Tomkins assumed that human beings are intrinsically motivated to maximize positive affect and to minimize negative affect. Any behavior that regularly evokes positive affect or reduces negative

affect will be consistently reinforced and thus more likely to be repeated. Because smoking has both stimulating and tension-reducing effects, it is likely to develop into a strong and persistent habit. To account for addictive smoking, Tomkins (1966) advanced the additional hypothesis that as dependence develops, the addictive smoker experiences "deprivation negative affect" as soon as he or she becomes aware of not smoking. This experience would be independent of feeling good or feeling bad at any particular moment.

Eysenck (1965, 1980) derived the diathesis–stress model of smoking from his general theory of personality. This could be seen as complementary to Tomkins' model, because it links smoking to cortical arousal and individual differences (Spielberger 1986). Research on the relationship between smoking and personality tends to provide evidence that smoking is weakly related to *extroversion*, *neuroticism* and *psychoticism*, the three dimensions of Eysenck's personality theory.

The diathesis–stress model suggests that people smoke for different reasons and that their motives for smoking are determined by their personality: extroverts have lower cortical arousal than introverts and frequently search for stimulation to heighten arousal. They should therefore smoke out of boredom in situations lacking in stimulation in order to increase their cortical arousal to a more optimal level. Eysenck further speculated that extroverts might smoke to conform to the behavior of their peers, because they are very dependent on social reinforcements.

Nicotine is a complex drug that acts as a stimulant in small doses but as a depressant in large ones. Introverts, who typically attempt to lower their habitually high cortical arousal, could therefore be expected to smoke for "tranquillizing purposes", mostly during periods of stress. Individuals who are anxious and emotionally unstable (high neuroticism) are prone to respond with more intense emotional reactions to environmental stress than emotionally stable individuals. They would therefore also be expected to smoke a great deal in stressful situations. Because neuroticism and extroversion/introversion are independent dimensions, one would expect the highest rate of smoking in *stressful* situations from individuals who are both introverted and neurotic.

The relationship between psychoticism and smoking is attributed to the tendency of individuals high on this dimension to be "tough-minded", and more likely to engage in antisocial–rebellious behavior. For persons high in psychoticism, smoking should therefore bring reinforcements from peers for this non-conforming behavior (Spielberger 1986).

Pharmacological theories
Whereas the psychological models suggested by Tomkins and Eysenck can account for such antagonistic motives as smoking to reduce anxiety or to increase stimulation, they have little to say about the causes of addictive smoking. Pharmacological models, on the other hand, have identified specific agents, either in the cigarettes or generated during combustion, which could be responsible for dependency. According to the nicotine regulation model developed by Schachter and his colleagues (Schachter 1977, 1978; Schachter *et al.* 1977b), individuals smoke to regulate the level of nicotine in the internal milieu. Smoking is stimulated when the nicotine level falls below a certain set point.

Schachter and his colleagues tested this hypothesis in a series of innovative studies (Schachter 1977; Schachter *et al.* 1977a, 1977b). In their first study, they lowered the level of nicotine in cigarettes and found that long-term, heavy smokers increased their smoking by 25 per cent, light smokers only by 18 per cent (Schachter 1977). To examine whether these changes reflected a need to maintain an optimal level of nicotine in the blood, Schachter *et al.* (1977a) compared smoking levels in subjects who were chemically induced to excrete nicotine either at a very high or a very low rate. Most of the nicotine absorbed by an individual is chemically broken down, mainly in the liver, but a fraction of nicotine which escapes this process is eliminated as such in the urine. The rate of excretion of unchanged nicotine (an alkaloid) in the urine depends on the acidity of the individual's urine. During different weeks, subjects in this experiment took either substantial doses of placebo or of drugs that acidify the urine (e.g. vitamin C = ascorbic acid). The fact that subjects who took vitamin C increased their average cigarette smoking by roughly 15–20 per cent supported this hypothesis.

It is puzzling to find that smokers are not only convinced that smoking reduces stress, but that they also smoke more in stressful situations like parties, examinations, colloquia, stressful seminar presentations or when being administered painful electric shocks (Schachter *et al.* 1977a). Schachter and his colleagues reasoned that this belief is based on the fact that stress makes the urine more acidic and thus lowers the blood-nicotine level. Thus, cigarette smoking under stress serves the function of regulating serum nicotine. To test this assumption, Schachter et al. (1977a) conducted an experiment which independently manipulated levels of stress and acidity of urine. Consistent with the nicotine regulation model, exposure to a painful rather than a weak electric shock increased smoking in subjects who had been given a placebo, but not in subjects who had been given a pill that prevented their urine from acidifying.

Does smoking help smokers to reduce stress, to calm down or to improve their performance? It does indeed, but only when compared with smokers who are deprived of nicotine. Thus, while smoking high-nicotine rather than low-nicotine cigarettes smokers can take more painful electric shocks, are less irritated by airplane noise and do better at motor performance tasks (Schachter 1978). However, when the mood or performance of smokers who are permitted to smoke ad lib are compared with the mood or performance of control groups of non-smokers, a depressing fact emerges – smoking only improves the mood of smokers or their performance *to the level customary for non-smokers* (Schachter 1978). In other words, "the heavy smoker gets nothing out of smoking. He [sic] smokes only to prevent withdrawal" (Schachter 1978: 106).

Biobehavioral explanations of smoking

The conclusion that smokers only smoke to prevent nicotine withdrawal symptoms has been criticized by Pomerleau and Pomerleau (1989). These authors argued that an addiction interpretation cannot explain the fact that many stimuli which reliably increase the probability of smoking are unrelated to the time since the last cigarette was smoked. Thus the temptation to smoke is increased at the end of a meal, when drinking a cup of coffee or when put under intellectual demands (Shiffman 1982). Pomerleau and Pomerleau (1989) suggested that nicotine alters the availability in the organism of behaviorally active neuroregulators. Thus smoking can be used as a pharmacological "coping response", resulting in temporary improvements in affect or performance.

Leventhal and Cleary (1980) integrated the models of Tomkins and Schachter into a "multiple regulation model", which assumes that smokers smoke to regulate emotional states and that nicotine levels are being regulated because certain emotional states have become conditioned to them. The authors discuss various processes by which such conditioning might occur. For example, distress induced by drops in the nicotine level could combine with the distress induced by high irritability or poor performance on various tasks. By smoking to return to nicotine base level, smokers have the rewarding experience of improving performance or reducing irritability. Thus, externally and internally generated cues are assumed to gain control over fluctuation in emotional states. This model integrates the pharmacological and psychological assumptions into a coherent theory of smoking.

Helping people to stop

Clinical intervention programs

Most clinical approaches to smoking cessation are based on cognitive behavior theory. The techniques used include classical conditioning (aversion therapy), operant procedures (stimulus control, contingency management), self-management procedures and nicotine fading. Most recent work relies on multicomponent programs that combine several of these techniques (for reviews, see Lichtenstein and Danaher 1975; Lichtenstein 1982; Glasgow and Lichtenstein 1987; Schwartz 1987; Hall *et al.* 1990). The use of nicotine chewing-gum has proved effective in the treatment of more nicotine-dependent patients, particularly when combined with behavioral therapy (for a review, see Cepeda-Benito 1993).

Three kinds of stimuli have been used in aversion therapies: electric shock, imaginal stimuli and cigarette smoke itself. *Shock aversion* has been consistently ineffective (Lichtenstein and Danaher 1975), and the efficacy of imaginal aversion or *covert sensitization* has also been fairly low. In this latter procedure, smokers have first to imagine themselves preparing to smoke and then to experience nausea. As an escape–relief dimension, they then imagine themselves feeling better as they turn away and reject their cigarettes. Smokers are usually given training in this procedure in the laboratory and are then asked to carry it out in their natural environments. In his extensive review of the effectiveness of smoking cessation techniques, Schwartz (1987: 81) concluded that "the cessation rates were low when covert sensitization was used alone, and when covert sensitization was combined with other procedures, it added little to effectiveness". However, he suggested that covert sensitization might be useful as a maintenance technique.

Cigarette smoke as an aversive stimulus is used in *rapid smoking*, a clinical procedure in which subjects are instructed to smoke continually, inhaling every 6–8 seconds, until tolerance is reached. This results in a nicotine satiation, and an irritation of the mucous membrane and throat passages which reduces smoking pleasure. It is expected that this unpleasant experience will be cognitively rehearsed and thus have a long-term effect. According to early research that relied mainly on unverified self-reports, rapid smoking produced a nearly 50 per cent abstinence rate 3–6 months after treatment (Lichtenstein and Danaher 1975). More recent studies of rapid smoking which used biochemical verification of abstinence have produced lower abstinence rates (for a review, see Hall *et al.* 1990). In recent years, rapid smoking has typically been combined with other intervention techniques. Schwartz (1987), who reviewed 49 rapid smoking trials reported between 1968 and 1985, found that 17 per cent of the studies using rapid smoking alone produced abstinence rates of at least 33 per cent at 1 year follow-up, compared with 50 per cent for those which combined rapid smoking with other treatment procedures. (The corresponding median cessation rates were 21 and 30.5 per cent, respectively.) Thus, rapid smoking used in multicomponent programs seems to be reasonably effective. However, rapid smoking affects the heart–lung system and results in increases in heart rate, carboxyhemoglobin and blood-nicotine levels (Lichtenstein 1982). Therefore, the health of patients should be assessed carefully before rapid smoking is selected as a treatment procedure. Patients should also be monitored closely during treatment.

Operant procedures are designed to detect the environmental stimuli that control the smoking response (stimulus control) or to manipulate the consequences of this response (e.g. contingency contracting). *Stimulus control* techniques are based on the assumption that smoking has become linked to environmental and internal events which trigger the smoking response (e.g. finishing a meal and drinking coffee or alcohol). Various techniques to extinguish the control of these stimuli over smoking have been used. The effectiveness of stimulus control approaches to smoking *cessation* has not been impressive, but stimulus control may assist smokers to reduce their smoking (Lichtenstein and Danaher 1975; Schwartz 1987).

In *contingency contracting*, smokers agree with some agency (usually the therapist) on a set of rewards/punishments that will be enacted contingent on their behavior. For example, smokers may pay a sum of money to the therapist and have it returned when they succeed in cutting down. Schwartz (1987) reviewed 13 contingency contracting trials reported between 1967 and 1985, and found that 89 per cent of the studies had a 33 per cent abstinence rate at 6 month follow-up, as compared with 25 per cent at 1 year follow-up. (The corresponding median cessation rates were 46 and 27 per cent, respectively.) Schwartz (1987) concluded that contracting is quite successful during treatment or until the deposit is returned. However, once the contract has ended, many subjects regress because no techniques for maintenance have been provided.

It would be plausible that subjects who abstain from smoking because they feel bound by a contract, attribute their *not* smoking to this agreement. They would therefore be less likely to develop a sense of self-efficacy and the feeling of control over their smoking behavior that is necessary to maintain their abstinence at the end of therapy (Bandura 1986). They might also not be motivated to engage in the kind of negative re-evaluation of smoking that is likely in people who have to justify to themselves the stopping of the habit.

Self-management procedures, which are also implemented under professional supervision, include many behavioral techniques, such as (1) the monitoring and recording of one's own smoking behavior, (2) changes in the antecedent conditions and consequences of one's smoking, and (3) developing awareness of, and changing, the environmental conditions that elicit smoking responses (Hall *et al.* 1990). The most effective use of self-management procedures seems to be as part of multicomponent programs. Self-management procedures used alone have not produced results better than the generally expected rates of 20–30 per cent abstinence at follow-up (Hall *et al.* 1990).

Monitored *nicotine fading* is a procedure by which subjects monitor their daily tar and nicotine intake and try to reduce progressively their nicotine intake (Foxx and Brown 1979). It is a procedure that is particularly suitable when smokers who have failed to give up completely try to achieve at least a lasting reduction in their smoking rate (Lichtenstein 1982).

Most recent behavioral treatments of smoking use *multicomponent treatments* and include a variety of methods. For example, most of these programs employ self-management. In addition, they may use relaxation training, or contingency contracting (Spring *et al.* 1978). Some of these programs also make use of aversion procedures such as rapid smoking (e.g. Lando 1977; Best *et al.* 1978). Schwartz (1987) reported median cessation rates for multi-component treatment trials of 40 per cent at 1 year follow-up. Two-thirds of these trials had medians that reached 33 per cent. According to Schwartz (1987), the more successful multicomponent programs have used a greater number of treatment sessions, stronger maintenance components, and manuals that guide and instruct the subject on how to use self-control procedures.

In view of the important role of nicotine dependence in smoking (Schachter 1978), it would seem useful to provide smokers with nicotine in the form of a chewing-gum (i.e. *nicotine gum*), at least as long as they are in the process of stopping. Once people have managed to stop smoking, withdrawal from the gum can be dealt with separately. There is evidence that gum treatment is very effective in helping people to stop (e.g. Russell *et al.* 1976; Harackiewicz *et al.* 1987). In a meta-analysis of 33 studies which employed nicotine chewing-gum in smoking treatment programs, Cepeda-Benito (1993) concluded that nicotine gum consistently improved the efficacy of *intensive* smoking cessation therapy and that it was the more effective the heavier people smoked. The superiority of intensive therapy plus nicotine gum over mere therapy was illustrated by the greater mean abstinence rates at long-term follow-up displayed by the nicotine gum groups (35 per cent) versus the control groups (22 per cent). Nicotine gum improved the overall effectiveness of intensive therapy by 56 per cent (Cepeda-Benito 1993).

Can cognitive behavior therapy, then, help smokers to maintain long-term abstinence? The answer seems to be a qualified "yes". Although there is considerable variability in outcomes across studies, replicable cognitive-behavioral intervention programs produce abstinence rates of 25–40 per cent at long-term follow-up. In particular, multicomponent treatment programs appear to be very effective. However, there is consistent evidence that heavy smokers who smoke more than 20 cigarettes a day are less likely to be successful (Glasgow and Lichtenstein 1987). Unfortunately, these are the persons most at risk of premature morbidity and mortality and therefore in particular need of treatment.

Community approaches to smoking control

Despite the substantial decline in cigarette smoking observed since the US Surgeon General's first report linking smoking to cancer, one cannot be confident that the decrease was not caused by some other factor (see Figure 3.1). To demonstrate the effectiveness of mass communication in inducing smoking cessation, we need *experimental* studies, in which one group of people is exposed to the communication while an otherwise comparable group is not. If it can be shown that the experimental group has an advantage in cessation rates over the control group, this difference can be attributed to the communication. Fortunately, such data are available from several major community studies which attempted to reduce smoking rates as part of their campaign to reduce the risk of coronary heart disease.

In one of his more recent reports, the US Surgeon General (1984) summarized the findings of community studies on smoking cessation (Table 4.1). Probably the most successful community intervention was achieved in the North Karelia Project described in the preceding chapter (e.g. Puska *et al.* 1985). As part of this project, an intensive educational campaign was implemented for the reduction of cigarette smoking. The neighboring province of Kuopio was selected as a control group not exposed to the campaign. Self-reported numbers of cigarettes smoked per day fell by more than one-third among the men in North Karelia, compared with only a 10 per cent reduction among the men in the control community. The campaign had no effect on the smoking rates of women. Although self-reports of smoking rates could be distorted by social desirability effects, it is encouraging that a 24 per cent decline in cardiovascular deaths was observed in North Karelia as compared with a 12 per cent decline in other parts of the country (Puska *et al.* 1985).

In the Stanford Three-Community-Study, only the experimental group which received face-to-face, intensive instruction in addition to the media exposures achieved a significant reduction when compared with the control group (Farquhar *et al.* 1977). Two other community studies conducted in Australia (Egger *et al.* 1983) and Switzerland (Autorengruppe Nationales Forschungsprogramm 1984) achieved a net reduction of 8–15 per cent. The US Surgeon General (1984) concluded that a reduction of 12 per cent in smoking rate was usual in this type of community intervention.

When compared with the 30 per cent success rate of the average therapy program, a 12 per cent reduction achieved by the much more cost-effective community interventions appears to be an acceptable rate. However, this may not be a fair comparison.

Table 4.1   Reduction in smoking observed in major community studies

Study	Years of study	Net per cent reduction in smoking[a]
Stanford Three-Community-Study	3	15–20
Australian North Coast Study	3	15
Swiss National Research Program	3	8
North Karelia Project	10	25[b]
Other large-scale studies[c]	2–10	5–25

[a] Difference between per cent reduction in proportion of smokers in the maximum intervention versus control conditions.
[b] Difference between per cent reduction in the mean number of cigarettes smoked per day among men.
[c] Clinical and worksite trials, the London Civil Servants Smoking Trial, the Göteborg Study, the Oslo Study, the WHO Collaborative Trial and the Multiple Risk Factor Intervention Trial.
Source: Adapted from US Surgeon General (1984).

Therapy programs probably have to deal with the hard-core smokers, those who have been unable or unwilling to give up their habit without outside help. A study conducted by Schachter (1982) supports the assumption that individuals who attempt to stop by themselves have less difficulty than those attending formal programs. Schachter interviewed the members of his own psychology department and a sample of people who worked in a small town in Long Island. He found that more than 60 per cent of the smokers who had attempted to stop had done so without outside help. Similar results were published by Rzewnicki and Forgays (1987).

However, the apparently greater ease of quitting smoking by people who have attempted it unaided could be an artifact: lifetime reports of successful stopping reflect success on one of a number of multiple attempts that have been made over the years. The evaluation of formal programs, on the other hand, reflects the success rate for a single trial. Because the probability of success increases with the number of attempts aggregated into a measure, higher success rates should be expected with measures reflecting repeated rather than single trials.

A comparison of rates on single trials for program participants and people who tried to give up by themselves, conducted by

Cohen and colleagues (1989), supported the latter interpretation. In contrast to Schachter's results, Cohen and his colleagues found that the cessation rates of smokers who stopped unaided were lower than those of smokers who attended formal programs. However, the success rates among self-quitters observed by Cohen *et al.* (1989) could have been unusually low. Their subjects were recruited from people who had called the American Lung Association or the American Cancer Association for self-help materials that had been advertised. This procedure could have resulted in an over-representation of hard-core smokers who had previously failed when trying to stop unaided.

Interventions at the worksite

As mentioned in Chapter 3, the place of work is an excellent setting for health promotion programs because large numbers of people can be reached on a regular basis. Furthermore, powerful incentives can be introduced to encourage healthy behavior. Therefore, many large firms have introduced health promotion programs. There is now growing evidence that these programs can be quite effective in helping individuals to stop smoking (for reviews, see Klesges and Glasgow 1986; Fielding 1991; Grunberg 1991).

Probably the best-known worksite health program is the Johnson and Johnson "Live for Life" (Wilbur *et al.* 1986; Fielding 1991). The major components of the Johnson and Johnson program are a health screen, a lifestyle seminar which introduces employees to the "Live for Life" concept, and a variety of health behavior improvement programs such as smoking cessation, exercise, stress management and nutrition, weight control, and general health knowledge. In addition, the company established a policy concerning smoking at the worksite.

A comparison of health indicators of the employees of Johnson and Johnson plants that participated in the program with the employees of plants that did not, revealed significantly higher smoking cessation rates for participating plants than for control plants (23 *vs* 17 per cent) over a 2 year period. These rates were based on self-reports and verified by biological measures (blood thiocyanate). The cessation rate difference was even higher for employees at high risk for coronary heart disease (32 *vs* 13 per cent).

A promising procedure which could be widely implemented in worksite health programs has been the institution of intergroup competitions to motivate individuals to adopt positive health behavior (e.g. Klesges *et al.* 1986, 1987). The effectiveness of this procedure has been demonstrated by Klesges and colleagues (1986), who evaluated worksite smoking cessation programs both with and without formal competition for monetary prizes in five financial institutions. The participants from the one worksite assigned to basic treatment received a 6 week cognitive-behavioral program that has been successfully implemented in both worksite and clinic settings. The employees in the four competition worksites received the same program. In addition, the presidents of these four institutions challenged each other at a press conference to see which site could produce the greatest reduction in smoking among its employees and success rates were compared continuously.

The findings indicate that the competition improved the effectiveness of the basic treatment. A greater percentage of employees who were smokers participated in the program with the competition than in the program without the competition (88 *vs* 53 per cent). Furthermore, although treatment outcome among the participants was generally equivalent at the end of the treatment (20 *vs* 30 per cent abstinence), at 6 month follow-up somewhat fewer participants in the basic treatment condition were still abstinent than in the competition condition (14 *vs* 18 per cent). Overall, the competition condition had a greater impact on smoking rates than the non-competition condition: 16 per cent of all smokers quit smoking in the competition condition, compared with 7 per cent in the worksite that received only the basic treatment. Furthermore, at 6 month follow-up, the subjects in the competition condition who were not abstinent had lower levels of carbon monoxide (an indicator of amount smoked) than subjects in the non-competition condition. These findings suggest that the competition was more effective in achieving abstinence or a reduction in smoking rates than was the basic treatment without competition.

Physicians' advice

Physicians can be important agents in health promotion. There is evidence that even minimal advice from physicians can be effective in changing smoking behavior. A classic study was conducted by Russell *et al.* (1979) in five group practices in London. During a 4 week period, 2138 cigarette smokers attending the medical practice of 28 general practitioners were assigned to one of four groups: (1) follow-up only; (2) questionnaire assessing their smoking behavior and follow-up; (3) physician's advice to stop smoking plus questionnaire and follow-up; and (4) advice to stop plus a leaflet helping them to stop and follow-up. Outcomes were assessed at 1 and 12 months and were biochemically validated.

The minimal intervention was quite effective. Compared with the non-intervention groups, more patients in the groups that received advice were successful in stopping after 1 year. In the two non-intervention groups, the proportion of patients who gave up smoking during the first months and were still not smoking 1 year later was 0.3 and 1.6 per cent for Groups 1 and 2, respectively. In comparison, 3.3 per cent of the patients who had merely been told to give up smoking and 5.1 per cent of the patients who in addition had received a leaflet with advice were still not smoking 1 year later. These differences may seem small but, as the authors argued, if all general practitioners in the UK were to adopt this procedure, the yield would exceed half a million ex-smokers within 1 year.

Primary prevention

School-based health education

In view of the serious difficulties smokers experience when they try to stop smoking, school-based anti-smoking programs aimed at preventing young adolescents from starting the habit would appear most promising. However, most of the early programs, which were conducted in health education courses and emphasized the long-term health risks of smoking, were ineffective in persuading children not to smoke (Thompson 1978). The likely reason for this failure is that children were already familiar with the health consequences of smoking and in any case are not yet very much concerned about health issues.

Programs developed by Evans and co-workers therefore avoided the health and threat-oriented approach that was predominant in earlier programs (e.g. Evans 1976: Evans et al. 1978). Instead, they emphasized the socially undesirable aspects of smoking to motivate individuals not to smoke (e.g. cigarettes smell bad). They also included the development of specific action plans and social skills to resist pressures to try cigarettes. Thus, individuals were trained in skills needed to reject offers of cigarettes without alienating peers.

In a review of four generations of school-based anti-smoking studies, only moderate reductions in the number of students who start smoking have been found (Flay 1985). Cleary and colleagues (1988) estimated that on average only 5–8 per cent of students who might otherwise have started to smoke were prevented from doing so. There is little evidence about the long-term effectiveness of such programs (Flay 1985).

The moderate success of school-based programs could be due to their focus on children who have not yet smoked any cigarettes. They may therefore be ineffective in reducing the likelihood that adolescents who have already experimented with cigarettes will become regular smokers. Leventhal et al. (1988) developed an anti-smoking program that incorporated measures which were aimed at slowing or reversing the progression from experimental to regular smoker. Their sessions focused on the experiences people have when they smoke their first few cigarettes. Their participants were told to interpret reactions such as coughing as signals of the body warning system not to smoke. It was pointed out that the disappearance of these signals was due to the body's warning system having been "knocked out" and did not mean that there were no negative health consequences from continued smoking. These authors presented data from a pilot study suggesting that students in their intervention groups were indeed less likely to progress from experimental to regular smokers (Hirschman and Leventhal 1989).

Legal and economic measures

A second strategy of primary prevention might involve further restrictions in the sales of cigarettes (e.g. stricter age limits) as well as increases in taxation. On average, teenagers have less disposable income than adults, and are therefore more likely to be deterred from smoking by marked increases in the price of cigarettes, particularly if they have not yet started the habit or are still in a period of experimentation. The price elasticity of demand for cigarettes varies from −1.40 in adolescents to −0.42 in adults (Lewit and Coate 1982). Thus, a 10 per cent increase in the price of cigarettes would result in a 14 per cent decrease in the demand for cigarettes among adolescents, but only in a 4 per cent decrease among adults.

On the basis of elasticity estimates such as these, Harris (1982) predicted that the 1982 doubling of the excise tax on cigarettes by the US Congress would result in a 3 per cent decline in the number of adult smokers but a 15 per cent decline among teenagers. This would remove 1.5 million adults and 700,000 adolescents from the high-risk cohort of smokers (Walsh and Gordon 1986). Because this doubling of the tax only involved a rise from 8 to 16 cents, more marked tax increases would seem a promising strategy to prevent young people from being recruited into smoking, particularly if these were combined with the various educational programs described earlier.

Conclusions

Smoking has been identified as the single most important source of preventable morbidity and mortality and nowadays this fact is accepted by smokers and non-smokers alike. Most smokers admit that they would like to stop. Although the rate of success of smokers who seek therapy is not always impressive, recent multicomponent treatment programs appear to have been quite effective. Furthermore, it has to be remembered that people who seek therapy are usually the most problematic cases.

Reasonable abstinence rates can also be achieved by minimal interventions such as community-based interventions, worksite programs or advice from physicians. Many smokers even seem to be able to stop without any help. Thus, surveys conducted by Schachter (1982) and Rzewnicki and Forgays (1987) suggested that approximately 60 per cent of smokers who had attempted to stop had succeeded at the time of the interview. These latter results are consistent with epidemiological data which indicate that the significant reduction in smoking rates observed during the last decades has been largely due to people who stopped unaided. However, giving up a long-established habit like smoking is always difficult. Therefore, the most promising strategy for smoking prevention would involve inducing people not to start smoking.

Alcohol and alcohol abuse

Alcohol and health

There is widespread consensus among health professionals that the inappropriate or excessive use of alcohol leads to an increased risk of morbidity and mortality (Bruun *et al.* 1975; Malin *et al.* 1982; Ashley and Rankin 1988; Hurley and Horowitz 1990). Ashley and Rankin (1988: 234) even claimed that "in the United States in 1977, total alcohol-related health costs ranked a close second to heart and vascular disease, as the prime health cause of economic loss, well ahead of cancer and respiratory disease". In recognition of these health risks, any alcoholic beverage that is bottled for sale in the USA now has to carry the following health warning:

Government Warning: According to the Surgeon General, women should not drink alcoholic beverages during pregnancy because of the risk of birth defects. Consumption of alcoholic beverages impairs your ability to drive a car or operate machinery, and may cause health problems.

The following section will review epidemiological evidence to document the health risk of excessive alcohol consumption.

Morbidity and mortality
Heavy drinkers suffer an increased risk of liver diseases (particularly cirrhosis), elevated blood pressure and various forms of cancer. Furthermore, the use and abuse of alcohol not only increases the likelihood of being involved in accidents, it has also been shown to increase the risk of serious injury to accident victims (Committee on Trauma Research 1985).

In the USA, only about 3 per cent of recorded deaths are officially attributed to causes directly linked to alcohol (Hurley and Horowitz 1990). However, epidemiologists suspect that there is a substantial under-reporting of alcohol-related conditions, particularly as contributing causes of death, and that the actual number is much higher (Hurley and Horowitz 1990).

One strategy to trace the relationship between mortality and excess alcohol consumption has been to demonstrate that the mortality rate of alcoholics for a given cause is in excess of that for moderate drinkers or abstainers (Bruun *et al.* 1975). However, in order to attribute a difference in mortality between these groups to the difference in alcohol consumption, one has to be certain that differential consumption is the only risk factor in which the two groups differ. This assumption is often unfounded, because people who are heavy drinkers or alcoholics usually engage in other habits that are deleterious to their health. For example, a review of studies on the relationship between alcoholism and smoking found that on average 90 per cent of the men and women in the alcoholic groups were smokers, a proportion that is much higher than that in the general population (Istvan and Matarazzo 1984). Thus, in interpreting findings that alcoholics suffer from an excess mortality from certain forms of cancer, one has to separate the impact of alcohol from that of smoking. For example, the excess cancer of the oral cavity, pharynx, larynx and esophagus among alcoholics must be attributed to the combined effects of both alcohol consumption and smoking (Bruun *et al.* 1975).

Alcohol and cirrhosis of the liver

A second strategy in investigating the health risk of alcohol abuse has been to focus on mortality from specific causes that are likely to be related to excess alcohol consumption. Not surprisingly, the most clear-cut evidence comes from mortality from cirrhosis of the liver. Cirrhosis is a disorder of the liver in which healthy liver tissue has at some time been damaged and replaced by fibrous scar tissue. In 1964, cirrhosis of the liver was the eleventh leading cause of death in the USA, and the fifth leading cause of death among men aged 25–64 years (Terris 1967). There is evidence of a positive correlation between per capita consumption of alcoholic beverages (measured in liters of absolute alcohol during a given year) and deaths due to liver cirrhosis (per 100,000 population aged 25 years and older). The data presented in Figure 4.1 show a correlation of 0.94 between these two variables across different nations (Schmidt 1977).

There is also evidence to suggest that restrictions imposed on alcohol consumption are accompanied by a fall in the number of deaths due to cirrhosis of the liver (Ledermann 1964). For example, in Paris there was a sharp drop in cirrhosis death rates coincidental with the two world wars. The data for the Second World War are particularly instructive, because cirrhosis deaths fell from 35 in 1941 to a low of 6 in 1945 and 1946. They began to rise again in 1948, the year when wine rationing was discontinued. Obviously, there were other factors present during this period that are likely to have at least contributed to the drop in liver cirrhosis mortality.

Alcohol and violent deaths

Alcohol has also been implicated in death from injuries. According to some estimates, a third to a half of adult Americans involved

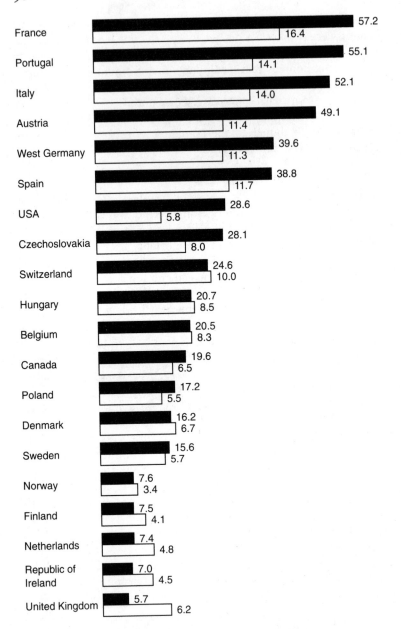

Figure 4.1 The relationship between per capita consumption of alcohol [in litres of absolute alcohol] (□) and death from cirrhosis of the liver [per 100, 000 population aged 25 and older] (■). *r* = 0.94
Source: Schmidt (1977)

Table 4.2   Blood or brain alcohol concentration for suicide, homicide and accident victims[a]

Casualty	Sample Size (n)	Per cent BAC = 0.10 and above	Per cent positive BAC
Suicide	247	16	32
Homicide	499	27	42
Motor vehicle			
driver	61	38	52
passenger	25	16	24
pedestrian	61	21	30
Fall	54	41	48
Fire	28	46	54
Drowning	19	53	68

[a] Data collected between 1974 and 1975.
Source: Adapted from Haberman and Baden (1978).

in accidents, crimes and suicides had been drinking alcohol prior to the event (Hurley and Horowitz 1990). At the same time, critics of these estimates have pointed out methodological weaknesses of the research and the tremendous range in the magnitude of the estimated involvement of alcohol in these violent deaths (e.g. Roizen 1982).

One major problem with research in this area is that it often lacks appropriate control groups. For example, in a very thorough study of the role of alcohol in violent deaths, Haberman and Baden (1978) report estimates of alcohol presence at the time of death for a sample of unnatural deaths that occurred in New York City between August 1974 and August 1975. Table 4.2 indicates the percentage of individuals in each event category for whom the presence of alcohol in the bloodstream could be demonstrated or who were intoxicated [a blood alcohol concentration (BAC) of more than 0.10 per cent].

Nevertheless, the fact that 52 per cent of the drivers killed in car accidents had previously consumed some alcohol is difficult to interpret unless we know the percentage of drivers of the same age and sex and with the same amount of alcohol at the same time and day who were not involved in accidents. If 52 per cent of those drivers had also consumed alcohol, there would be no case to argue that alcohol consumption increases the risk of traffic accidents. However, the evidence from studies that employed adequate control groups suggests that alcohol consumption significantly increases the risk of injuries from all types of accidents. In a study of drivers that were killed in car accidents in New York City, McCarroll and Haddon (1962) found that 50 per cent had a BAC at or above the 0.10 per cent level (i.e. were fairly intoxicated), compared with less than 5 per cent of drivers tested at the site of the accident a few weeks later. These tests were conducted on the same day of week and at the same time of day at which the accident had occurred, with drivers moving in the same direction. Similarly, a study of fatally injured adult pedestrians that used the same type of control group reported that 74 per cent of those injured had consumed some alcohol, compared with 33 per cent of those in the control group (Haddon et al. 1961). Taken together, these studies strongly suggest that people who have consumed alcohol are at an increased risk of accidental injuries and violent death.

Is there a protective effect of moderate consumption?
In view of the high proportion of smokers among alcoholics, it is surprising that studies of the impact of alcohol consumption on coronary death often find no relationship (e.g. Dawber 1980), or even the positive relationship that moderate drinkers have lower mortality rates than abstainers (e.g. Hennekens et al. 1979). The existence of an apparently protective association between light-to-moderate alcohol consumption and coronary heart disease has recently been questioned by Shaper et al. (1988). These authors concluded from a prospective study of more than 7000 middle-aged men that the apparently positive health impact of moderate drinking is a selection artifact: men who have health problems reduce their drinking and thus move into the non-drinking or occasional drinking category. However, a large case-control study conducted in New Zealand compared the risk among light and moderate drinkers with that of life-long abstainers and found that drinking up to five to six drinks a week was associated with a reduced risk of myocardial infarction (Jackson et al. 1991). Further research is needed to reconcile these contradictory findings.

Fetal alcohol syndrome
Aristotle was probably the first to observe that drunken women often bore children who were feeble-minded. However, the advice

of the US Surgeon General for women not to drink alcohol during pregnancy is based on more recent observations suggesting that prenatal exposure to alcohol is associated with a distinct pattern of birth defects that have been termed the fetal alcohol syndrome (FAS). A number of physical malformations have been reported; for example, head circumference and nose are smaller, the nasal bridge is lower, there is a growth deficiency. However, the most serious aspect of the FAS is mental retardation (Abel 1980). Although the exact number of children born with this syndrome is not known, it is estimated that in the USA one to two live-births per 1000 (or 4000–5000 births per year) are afflicted.

Although the description of the FAS is non-controversial, its causes and the level of alcohol consumption during pregnancy that is considered safe are highly disputed. Women who drink excessively during pregnancy are also likely to do a number of other things that are unhealthy to the fetus, such as smoking, not eating properly and even taking drugs. For example, nutritional deficiencies during pregnancy could actually be responsible for the low birthweight of the children born with FAS. However, as Logue (1986) concluded, the evidence now strongly suggests that alcohol is directly responsible. Current estimates place the fetus at risk for the physical signs of FAS if maternal drinking during pregnancy is six glasses of wine per day (450 ml of wine or approximately 60 ml of absolute alcohol) (Abel 1980).

Hazardous consumption levels and alcoholism

What level of consumption is hazardous to the health of men (or non-pregnant women)? This is largely a matter of conjecture. Clark and Midanik (1982) defined a heavy drinker as one who ingests 30 ml or more of pure alcohol a day (one ounce or more). Thus somebody who drinks three or more drinks would already be considered a heavy drinker. It should be noted that three glasses of wine per day at 75 ml of wine per glass contain approximately 30 ml of pure alcohol.

Approaching the problem from the standpoint of the lower limit of consumption of clinical alcoholics, Schmidt and de Lint (1970) found that the reported consumption of 96 per cent of the alcoholics in their sample was a daily intake at or above 150 ml of pure alcohol, the quantity of alcohol contained in one liter of Burgundy. There is reason to doubt the accuracy of such self-reports, however,

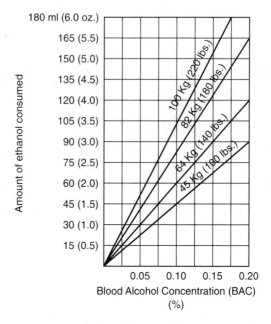

Figure 4.2   Nomogram of ethanol (pure alcohol) intake, body weight and blood alcohol concentration (from Mooney 1982). *Note*: To approximate the BAC, trace horizontally to the right to intercept the diagonal line representing body weight. Then trace downward to find the peak BAC. This process can be reversed to estimate the amount of alcohol consumed. The BAC falls consistently at 0.015 per cent per hour

because representative surveys done in the USA, Finland and Canada on self-reported consumption account for only 40–50 per cent of total alcohol sales when projected to the whole population (Furst 1983).

However, even if accurate, measures of the quantity of drinking are of little help in diagnosing alcoholism. As Vaillant (1983: 22) pointed out, "a yearly intake of absolute alcohol that would have represented social drinking for the vigorous 100-kilogram Winston Churchill with his abundant stores of fat would spell medical and social disaster for an epileptic woman of 60-kilograms or for an airline pilot with an ulcer". Thus the percentage of pure alcohol in an individual's blood (the BAC) which is used by governments all over the world to determine safe driving limits, depends very much on body weight (Figure 4.2).

A more promising approach to the definition of alcohol abuse, and one that is more in line with the common view of alcoholism, is to combine reported consumption and reported problems related to drinking (Furst 1983). Thus, the *Diagnostic and Statistical Manual of Mental Disorders* (DSM-III-R; American Psychiatric Association 1987) defines *alcohol abuse* according to two broadly defined categories: (1) pathological use (e.g. need for daily use, inability to cut down or stop, binges and blackouts) and (2) impairment in social and occupational functioning (e.g. job loss, legal difficulties, belligerence while drinking). These symptoms must have been present for at least 1 month.

The DSM-III-R also distinguishes alcohol abuse from alcohol dependence, the latter being the more serious form of alcoholism. The alcohol-dependent person is one who, in addition to some of the above symptoms of alcohol abuse, shows evidence that he or she has tolerance to the effects of alcohol or has experienced withdrawal symptoms. Using these criteria, a community study conducted between 1981 and 1983 in the USA indicated that approximately 13 per cent of the adult population were alcohol-dependent or alcohol abusers at some time in their lives (American Psychiatric Association 1987: 174).

Theories of alcohol abuse

Theories of alcohol abuse can be divided into two groups: (1) those that view it as an identifiable unitary disease process, and (2) those that conceive it in terms of behavioral models. This section will discuss both these approaches.

The disease concept of alcohol abuse

Of the various disease conceptualizations of alcoholism which have appeared in the literature over the past 40 years (e.g. Alcoholics Anonymous 1955; Jellinek 1960), the one developed by Jellinek has become most widely known. Jellinek (1960) presented a typology of alcoholism, specifying two types of alcoholic disease, which he called the "gamma" and the "delta" syndromes. Gamma alcoholism, which is the predominant type of alcoholism in North America, is characterized by: (1) acquired increased tissue tolerance to alcohol; (2) adaptive cell metabolism; (3) physical dependence on alcohol (craving); and (4) loss of control. Once a person with gamma alcoholism begins to drink, he or she is unable to stop. The social damage is general and severe. In delta alcoholism, which is said to be the predominant type of alcoholism in France and other wine-drinking countries, the gamma alcoholic's inability to stop is replaced by an inability to abstain. Delta alcoholics drink great amounts of alcohol on a regular basis. There is little social or psychological damage, but there may be physical damage, such as cirrhosis of the liver.

It has been hypothesized that the difference between alcoholics and non-alcoholics is based on a psychological predisposition, an allergic reaction to alcohol, or some nutritional deficits which may or may not be genetically influenced (Caddy 1978). One major implication of this approach is that treatment must emphasize the permanent nature of the alcoholic's problem and that the disease can only be arrested by lifelong abstinence.

Despite a great deal of research, there is no reliable empirical evidence for a psychological predisposition (Vaillant 1983), nor for the physiological processes assumed by the disease model to lead to alcoholism (George and Marlatt 1983). Furthermore, there is now evidence that, rather than having to give up alcohol altogether, some alcoholics (the less severely dependent ones) can be taught to return to controlled social drinking through therapy (Lloyd and Salzberg 1975; Heather and Robertson 1983; Rosenberg 1993). Definitions of controlled drinking have varied but have usually included some limit on the amount and frequency of consumption (e.g. a maximum of 30 ml alcohol per day) and the condition that drinking results in neither signs of dependence nor social, legal or health problems (Rosenberg 1993).

Most damaging to Jellinek's conception, however, have been studies examining the "loss of control" hypothesis using balanced placebo designs (Maisto *et al.* 1977; Marlatt *et al.* 1973; Berg *et al.* 1981). These studies examined the hypothesis that the apparent "loss of control" after alcohol consumption is due to the *knowledge* that one has consumed alcohol rather than to the pharmacological effects of alcohol. The knowledge that they have drunk alcohol probably provides subjects with an excuse to consume more alcohol. The balanced placebo design allows one to manipulate independently expected and actual beverage content.

For example, social drinkers and alcoholics who participated in the study of Marlatt *et al.* (1973), were either led to believe that their drinks would contain vodka and tonic, or that it would contain only tonic. In fact, half the subjects in each of those conditions received a drink containing vodka, the other half receiving tonic water only. Following this drink, the subjects had to participate in a taste-rating of alcoholic beverages. Those subjects who believed that their "primer" drink had contained alcohol drank significantly more than subjects who expected only tonic. The amount consumed was unaffected by the actual alcohol content of these drinks, thus disconfirming the loss of control hypothesis.

Furthermore, studies using the balanced placebo design suggest that many of the behavioral consequences of alcohol are due to expectations about the effects of alcohol rather than its pharmacological impact (Marlatt *et al.* 1973; Marlatt and Rohsenow 1980; Hull and Bond 1986). In particular, the knowledge that one has consumed alcohol appears to disinhibit enjoyable but illicit behavior (such as sexual behavior or further alcohol consumption) by providing an excuse for what would otherwise be considered inappropriate acts (Hull and Bond 1986).

Genetics and alcoholism

It is ironic that at a time when Jellinek's disease model seemed to have been thoroughly discredited, research into the heredity of drinking habits and into biological markers for alcoholism produced evidence suggesting some form of biological vulnerability to alcoholism (for reviews, see Hill *et al.* 1986; Devor and Cloninger 1989; Hurley and Horowitz 1990). Although it had long been known that susceptibility to alcoholism runs in families, it seemed reasonable to attribute this relationship to socialization rather than heredity. Studies have shown that the sons of alcoholics are several times more likely to become alcoholics than are the sons of non-alcoholics (e.g. Goodwin *et al.* 1973). For example, Goodwin and colleagues (1973) compared the drinking habits of 55 male adoptees with an alcoholic biological parent with that of 78 control adoptees without such a history. They found that 18 per cent of the adoptees with an alcoholic parent compared with 5 per cent of the controls developed alcohol problems. Thus, the adoptees whose biological parents had been alcoholics were more than three times as likely themselves to become alcoholic in adult life.

Even more surprising, when Goodwin *et al.* (1974) compared adopted-away sons of alcoholics with their own brothers who had been raised by the alcoholic biological parent, the rates of alcoholism turned out to be rather similar in the two groups. As Goodwin *et al.* (1974: 168) concluded: "sons of alcoholics were no more likely to become alcoholic if they were reared by their alcoholic parent than if they were separated from their alcoholic parent soon after birth and reared by non-relatives". Comparable results were reported by Bohman (1978). Furthermore, Bohman *et al.* (1981) presented evidence that suggested maternal inheritance of alcoholism in women. They reported a three-fold excess of alcohol abusers among women who were born to alcoholic mothers but were adopted during the first few months of life by non-relatives.

. The children in these studies had been separated from their alcoholic biological parents, and thus from any predisposing environmental influence arising from an alcoholic home, before the age of 3 and in most cases during the first few months of life. The predominant environmental influence therefore came from their adoptive homes. And yet, they were more than three times as likely to develop alcohol problems. These findings therefore strongly support the hypothesis that genetic factors contribute to susceptibility to alcoholism. It is important to note, however, that they do not imply that the development of alcoholism is *unaffected* by environmental factors. They merely indicate that the environment provided by an alcoholic parent does not increase the risk of alcoholism. This may seem puzzling at first, but it has to be considered that having an alcoholic parent may also serve as a salient and very effective reminder of the negative consequences of excessive drinking.

The evidence suggesting a genetic susceptibility led to an increased search for biological markers of alcoholism – that is, for indicators which allow one to identify those individuals who are vulnerable, regardless of whether they have ever displayed alcoholic behavior or even heavy drinking. Recent neurophysiological studies have recorded electrical potential from the scalp of subjects who were actively processing information during problem-solving tasks (so-called event-related-potentials or ERPs). They found a number of differences between first-degree relatives of alcoholics and individuals without such a family history (for a review, see Hill *et al.* 1986).

Thus, even though several of the specific hypotheses (e.g. loss of control) of the model of Jellinek (1960) have not been supported, his general assumption that there is a biological vulnerability to alcohol appears to be valid (Hill *et al.* 1986). It should be emphasized, however, that even if we accept the existence of some form of biological vulnerability, this does not mean that every individual who is vulnerable also develops alcohol problems or that only those who are vulnerable develop them. The vulnerability conception merely implies that some individuals are at a slightly greater risk for alcoholism due to a biological precondition.

Behavioral models of alcohol abuse

Behavioral approaches to understanding the causes and development of alcohol abuse subsume a number of diverse conceptual models that share the common emphasis on learning processes. According to this approach, alcoholism is fundamentally a manner of drinking alcohol that has either been learned through conditioning (classical, operant) or through observational learning. Because we cannot do justice to the whole range of behavioral theories of alcoholism within the context of this chapter, we will focus on the best-known learning theory of alcohol use and abuse, namely the Tension Reduction Hypothesis of alcohol consumption (Cappell and Greeley 1987). Some cognitive modifications of this model will also be discussed (e.g. Marlatt 1976; Hull 1981, 1987). The reader interested in a more extensive review and evaluation of psychological theories of alcoholism is referred to the excellent volume edited by Blane and Leonard (1987).

The basic assumption of the *tension reduction hypothesis* is that alcohol is consumed because it reduces tension. According to this model: (1) increased tension constitutes a heightened drive state; (2) by lowering tension and thus reducing this drive state, alcohol consumption has reinforcing properties; and (3) such drive-reducing reinforcement strengthens the alcohol consumption response.

Research conducted with animals and humans to test the original model has produced rather inconclusive findings (for reviews, see Cappell and Herman 1972; George and Marlatt 1983; Cappell and Greeley 1987). The major problem with the tension reduction hypothesis is the assumption of a linear relationship between alcohol consumption and tension reduction. Contrary to this assumption, experimental evidence indicates that alcohol produces a biphasic response, with small amounts leading to a state of arousal that is experienced by the drinker as a euphoric high. With continued consumption, this phase gives way to a suppressive effect accompanied by tension and depression (George and Marlatt 1983). This could explain most of the inconsistencies in research results.

More recently, two cognitive models have been developed which may be able to account for most of the inconsistencies in research that has tested the tension reduction hypothesis with human subjects (Hull 1981, 1987; George and Marlatt 1983). George and Marlatt (1983) argued that because the relaxing and euphoric effect associated with small amounts of alcohol immediately follows the initiation of drinking, it has a much more potent associative tie to drinking behavior than the delayed negative effect. Thus, people may drink to have this positive effect. George and Marlatt suggested that it is the expected rather than the actual tension-reducing properties of alcohol that are most influential in determining alcohol consumption. People drink because they expect that it will relax them.

In developing their cognitive model, George and Marlatt (1983) drew on the findings of McClelland *et al.* (1972) that the consumption of alcohol leads to increased fantasies of personal "power". George and Marlatt reasoned that if alcohol produced an increase in both physiological arousal and fantasies of personal power or control, drinking would increase in situations in which the drinker feels deprived of personal control. Lack of control is one of the major features that characterizes stressful situations (Seligman 1975).

George and Marlatt (1983) predicted that the probability of excessive or inappropriate drinking would vary as a function of the following variables: (1) the degree to which individuals exposed to a particular situation feel that they are helpless and have no control over their outcomes; (2) the availability of an adequate coping response as an alternative to drinking in such a high-risk situation; and (3) the person's expectation about the effectiveness of alcohol as an alternative coping response in the situation. Thus, if a drinker experiences a loss of personal control in a stressful situation and has no other adequate coping response available, the probability of drinking will increase. Under these conditions, alcohol consumption has the function of restoring the person's sense of personal control. George and Marlatt (1983) argued that this model offered a coherent explanation for most of the research testing the tension reduction hypothesis with human subjects.

Whereas Marlatt and colleagues see helplessness and the need for personal control as an important motive underlying problem drinking, Hull (1981, 1987) suggested that individuals consume alcohol to lower their level of self-awareness following failure, in order to avoid negative self-evaluation. Self-awareness is a state of self-focused attention in which individuals compare their real and their ideal self (Duval and Wicklund 1973). When such comparisons lead to unfavorable results (i.e. when the real self does not measure up to the ideal), negative affect is created. This motivates the individual to either reduce the self-ideal discrepancy or to avoid self-awareness. There is empirical evidence that alcohol interferes with encoding processes fundamental to a state of self-awareness, and thereby decreases the individual's sensitivity to both the self-relevance of cues regarding appropriate forms of behavior and the self-evaluative nature of feedback about past behavior (Hull et al. 1983). By lowering the individual's level of self-awareness, alcohol consumption decreases negative self-evaluation following failure.

Both Marlatt (1976; George and Marlatt 1983) and Hull (1981, 1987) emphasized that their models offer only a partial explanation of alcohol use and abuse. Thus, drinking is also likely to be affected by such factors as observational learning and social reinforcement in situations that are not stressful. There is also overlap in the conditions which should encourage problem drinking according to these two models. However, whereas failure situations tend to be stressful, not all stressful situations involve failure. Thus, the husband whose spouse has died of cancer may experience (universal) helplessness but not failure. And yet bereavement has been found to be associated with an increased risk of alcohol abuse, at least for men (for a review, see Stroebe and Stroebe 1987).

Behavioral treatment of alcohol problems

Virtually all approaches to the treatment of alcoholism include some behavioral treatment procedures (Caddy and Block 1983). Since excellent reviews of behavioral treatment procedures are available (e.g. Litman and Topham 1980; Caddy and Block 1983; Riley et al. 1987; Hurley and Horowitz 1990), we will give only a brief overview.

Treatment goals
With the increased acceptance of behavioral approaches to alcoholism, the goals of treatment have also changed. Although the proponents of Jellinek's disease concept believed that the only cure for alcoholism was complete abstinence, some behavior therapists

felt that at least the less severely dependent alcoholics could be taught to drink moderately. Several factors seem to be important in predicting which problem drinkers may succeed at controlled drinking rather than complete abstinence (for reviews, see Miller and Hester 1986; Rosenberg 1993). Individuals who have the best prospects are relatively young, married and are employed, and have had a relatively brief history of alcohol abuse, and believe that the goal of controlled drinking is attainable. Controlled drinking training does not seem to be an effective method for chronic alcoholics who are severely dependent. Once severe dependence has occurred, the alcoholic no longer has the option of returning to social drinking (Hurley and Horowitz 1990). Thus complete abstinence still appears to be the preferred goal for most patients who need clinical treatment.

Detoxification

Before the initiation of therapy, alcoholics frequently have to be "dried out". In severe cases, they may need medication to counteract alcohol withdrawal symptoms, which include anxiety, tremors and hallucinations. There are basically two approaches to detoxification. One method employs the substitution of alcohol with another more easily controlled drug in this category (usually barbiturates or benzodiazepines). A slow reduction of the medication minimizes withdrawal symptoms (Mooney and Cross 1988). An alternative approach uses minimal medication in the hope that severe withdrawal symptoms will help patients to recognize the severity of their condition. Obviously, the second approach requires very close medical supervision.

Clinical intervention programs

Depending on the noxious stimulus employed, three kinds of aversion therapy can be distinguished. *Electrical aversion therapy* pairs alcohol cues repeatedly with electric shock until a conditioned response (anxiety) is developed in response to these alcohol cues (cf. McGuire and Vallance 1964). Anxiety should then trigger alcohol avoidance, which is presumably reinforced by anxiety reduction. In *chemical aversion therapy*, patients who have been given an emetic (vomiting-inducing) drug are then administered alcohol a few minutes before nausea and vomiting occurs. Again it is hoped that the nausea response becomes associated with the alcohol cues (e.g. Wiens and Menustik 1983). Chemical aversion can also be induced by administering disulfiram, a drug that leads to nausea and vomiting whenever the patient drinks alcohol. Thus, alcoholics treated with the drug disulfiram are exposed to a taste aversion paradigm each time they drink alcohol. Finally, in *verbal aversion therapy* (covert sensitization), the noxious stimulus consists of aversive imagery which is repeatedly paired with alcohol-related imagery (Cautela 1966; Elkins 1980).

Contingency management involves arranging the individual's environment so that positive consequences follow desired behavior and either negative or neutral consequences follow undesirable behavior. Crucial to the planning of therapeutic strategies based on contingency management is the identification of reinforcers that maintain drinking behavior as well as the rewards that may be manipulated to modify the drinking. Because marital partners are important sources of reinforcement in everyday life, they have been included in designing therapy. Thus wives of alcohol abusers have been taught basic principles of behavior modification (Cheek *et al.* 1971) or have been involved in behavioral contracting between an alcohol abuser and his wife (Miller 1972). Other interesting applications of contingency management techniques have used behavioral contracting to increase participation in treatment programs or aftercare (e.g. Bigelow *et al.* 1976; Pomerleau *et al.* 1978).

Self-management procedures accept that individuals can arrange their own reinforcement contingencies in order to make certain behavior more likely (e.g. Miller and Munoz 1976; Miller *et al.* 1980). For example, they can reward themselves for doing something which is unpleasant or punish themselves for transgressing predetermined rules. The major components of self-management programs are: (1) self-monitoring of alcohol consumption; (2) functional analysis of drinking; (3) manipulating the antecedents and consequences of drinking; and (4) goal-setting. Self-monitoring of drinking usually reveals some regularities in the individual's drinking behavior. Individuals can reorganize their environments to avoid circumstances associated with heavy drinking. Goals may be negotiated which set precise limits to alcohol consumption (Miller and Munoz 1976).

Skill training procedures are based on the assumptions that (1) alcoholics lack certain skills to deal with their environments, and (2) that they use alcohol as an alternative coping strategy. For example, alcohol abusers frequently seem to drink as a coping response to stressful interpersonal situations (Miller *et al.* 1974; Higgins and Marlatt 1975). It is therefore plausible that interpersonal skill training should improve the individual's control over a potential stressor. Similarly, relaxation training may be given to improve the problem drinker's ability to deal with stressful situations. An even more extensive approach, the "Community Reinforcement Approach", includes problem-solving training, behavioral family therapy, social counselling and – for unemployed clients – job-finding training (Hunt and Azrin 1973; Azrin 1976). The importance of this type of skill training follows from the cognitive theories of George and Marlatt (1983) and Hull (1981), who conceive of stress and failure experiences as potent motivators of alcohol consumption.

Skill training is typically used as part of a broad-spectrum approach, which addresses life problems related to the drinking as well as drinking behavior (Lazarus 1965). In their careful evaluation of different methods of alcoholism treatment, Miller and Hester (1986: 154) draw the following conclusions:

> Current research provides sound support for at least three broad-spectrum approaches: social skills training, stress management training, and community reinforcement approach. All three involve training clients in specific coping skills. Initial data on differential improvement indicate that such training is of maximal benefit to clients who are deficient in these coping skills.

The *effectiveness* of the behavioral and non-behavioral treatment of alcohol abuse has been assessed extensively (e.g. Costello 1975a, 1975b; Litman and Topham 1980; Riley *et al.* 1987). Riley and colleagues (1987) evaluated 68 alcoholism treatment studies that were published between 1978 and 1983 in peer-reviewed English language publications, and which had follow-up periods of between 6 and 144 months. The outcomes of 30 studies (4894 subjects) which used behavioral treatment of alcoholism were as follows: Of the subjects who received treatment, 1 per cent were reported as being deceased, 16 per cent were lost to follow-up, 41 per cent were regarded as successes (i.e. moderating or terminating their drinking) and 40 per cent were regarded as failures (i.e. still drinking with an associated problem).

A comparison of outcome rates with those of 49 studies (9652 subjects) which used non-behavioral treatment procedures indicated that the two types of studies were similar with regard to subjects classified as failures. However, a slightly higher percentage of subjects receiving behavioral rather than non-behavioral treatment was reported as being successful (Riley *et al.* 1987). When the outcomes for both procedures were combined, the findings were similar to those reported by Costello (1975b) for studies conducted between 1951 and 1973.

Does behavioral treatment improve people's chances of overcoming their alcohol problem? One way to address this question is to compare treatment outcomes with the remission rates of untreated alcoholism. Only limited data are available on the rates of spontaneous remission (Kendell and Staton 1966; Imber *et al.* 1976; Polich *et al.* 1981). Polich and colleagues (1981) reported that of those treated alcoholics interviewed 4 years after treatment, 28 per cent had been abstinent for at least 6 months at the time of the interview, compared with 16 per cent of the untreated alcoholics. Imber *et al.* (1976), who conducted a follow-up study of 83 alcohol abusers who did not receive any treatment other than simple detoxification, reported an abstinence rate of 19 per cent for 1 year follow-up and 11 per cent for 3 year follow-up. The comparison of treated and untreated alcohlics is problematic for two reasons. On the one hand, individuals who enter therapy are likely to have more severe alcohol problems than those who do not; on the other hand, those who enter therapy may also be more motivated to stop drinking. However, the comparison does suggest that even though not all alcoholics require formal treatment for alcoholism in order to recover, those who enter clinical treatment have a slightly better chance of recovery, at least within the limits usually evaluated in treatment outcome follow-ups.

Primary prevention

Since the late 1960s, the attention of those concerned with public health aspects of alcohol has shifted from individuals suffering from alcoholism to the general overall consumption of alcohol in a given society and the factors that affect this consumption (Ashley and Rankin 1988). This change of approach was motivated by the research of Ledermann (1956, 1964). According to Lederman, the frequency distribution of drinkers in a population is continuous, unimodal and positively skewed (Figure 4.3). The fact that there

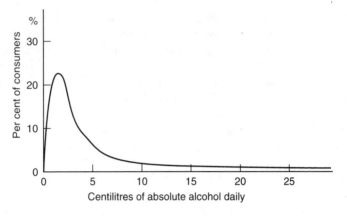

Figure 4.3 Frequency distribution of alcohol consumption
Source: de Lint (1977)

is no separate peak at the high end of the distribution for alcoholics suggests that (1) the proportion of heavy drinkers in a given
population can be estimated from knowledge of the mean per
capita consumption, and (2) that this proportion can be decreased
by reducing the mean per capita consumption by means of fiscal
and legal measures.

Consistent with Lederman's position, there is convincing evidence that per capita consumption and excessive drinking (inferred
from death rates due to cirrhosis of the liver) are closely related
(see Figure 4.1). Although one cannot infer causality on the basis
of only correlational evidence, the finding that restrictions imposed
on alcohol consumption led to a fall in the number of deaths due
to cirrhosis of the liver, suggests that measures reducing the per
capita consumption are likely to result in a decrease in alcohol
problems.

There are two main strategies of primary prevention which have
been employed to reduce drinking problems, namely, health protection measures aimed at controlling the availability of alcohol
and health education to persuade people not to engage in harmful
drinking. *Health protection measures* include legislative and regu-
latory controls of the price of beverages, numbers and locations of
outlets, hours and days of sale. Studies spanning several decades
have indicated that price control via taxation can be effective in
reducing alcohol consumption (Ashley and Rankin 1988; Hurley
and Horowitz 1990).

It has been demonstrated that the demand for alcoholic beverages responds to changes in price and income. For example, Johnson and Oksanen (1977), who used data on the relationship between changes in the price of alcoholic beverages and consumption in 10 Canadian provinces between 1956 and 1970, estimated the elasticity for beer at −0.29, for spirits at −1.70 and for wine at −1.36. According to these estimates, the demand for spirits and wine was more likely to respond to changes in price than that for beer.

On the basis of a quasi-experimental design, Cook (1981) came to very similar estimates of the elasticities in demand for spirits in the USA. He compared changes in the consumption of liquor in 39 US states before and after a significant rise in excise taxes with changes in the consumption for the same period in comparable states in which taxes had not been increased. In 30 of the 39 states, there was a decrease in consumption following the increase in taxation as compared with the comparison states. The price elasticity was estimated at −1.6, which implies that a 10 per cent increase in the price of spirits in a state resulted in a 16 per cent reduction in quantity purchased in that state. Cook (1981, 1982) argued that a doubling of federal tax on liquor in the USA would lead to a 20 per cent reduction in the nation's mortality from cirrhosis of the liver.

That price increases can also affect the drinking habits of heavy drinkers has been shown in a study of individual drinkers conducted in Scotland before and after a substantial increase in tax on alcoholic beverages (Kendell *et al.* 1983a, 1983b). It was found that alcohol consumption had fallen by 18 per cent after the tax increase and that this effect was at least as strong for heavy as for lighter drinkers. There was a similar reduction in the adverse effects of alcohol, such as getting into fights through drinking or being involved in a road accident after drinking. Participants were also aware that they had reduced their level of drinking since the last survey and the main reason offered was the increase in the price of alcohol. The authors concluded from their findings that increases in excise duty on alcoholic beverages can be an effective public health measure.

Health education programs have been shown to affect public knowledge about, and attitudes toward alcohol, but it has not been demonstrated convincingly that such programs have resulted in behavior change leading to a reduction in per capita consumption (Ashley and Rankin 1988). This is not too surprising, however, because these education programs are likely to be counteracted by the pervasive efforts of the alcohol industry in promoting alcohol consumption. For example, in 1981, an estimated US$2 billion was spent on alcoholic beverage advertising in the USA (Ashley and Rankin 1988).

Summary and conclusions

Alcoholism and alcohol abuse are now widely recognized as serious public health problems. Alcohol abuse is characterized by a long-standing pathological pattern of daily alcohol consumption, and an impairment of social or occupational functioning. Although there is a biological vulnerability to alcohol, drinking patterns are learnt and can be influenced by changes in reinforcement contingencies. However, in view of the moderate success rates of treatment techniques, strategies of health protection and health education that aim to prevent alcoholism would appear to be a necessary additional approach to reduce alcohol problems in society.

Eating control, overweight and obesity

Obesity is a medical problem that, like alcoholism, carries a social stigma. Society has a strong bias against people who are obese (Allon 1973), a bias that can even be found in young children (Maddox et al. 1968). But unlike people with physical handicaps, obese persons not only suffer the stigma of their obesity, they are also blamed for it. The common view holds that people are obese because they eat too much and that it is up to them to slim down. And yet the evidence on differences in food intake of obese and normal weight individuals is less than conclusive (Garrow 1974; Wooley et al. 1979; Striegel-Moore and Rodin 1986). Furthermore, results of treatment outcome studies suggest that obese individuals have great difficulty in reducing their weight even if they want to do so (Brownell 1982).

Overweight, obesity and bodyweight standards

The concepts of overweight and obesity imply a standard of normal or ideal weight against which a given weight is judged. Because height and weight are highly correlated, such a standard will have to be height-specific. One solution defines normal weight in terms of the average weight of large samples of persons representing the general population and characterized by sex, age and height. Instead of average weight, the metropolitan relative weight (MRW) uses the ideal weight as a reference point (i.e. the weight associated with the lowest mortality in insurance statistics). The MRW is computed for each subject by forming the ratio of his or her body weight and the ideal weight for his or her height (Simopoulos 1986). Overweight is defined as a body weight that is between the upper limit of normal and 20 per cent above that limit. A body weight that is more than 20 per cent above that limit would be considered obese (Bray 1986). Obesity has been further classified into mild (20–40 per cent), moderate (41–100 per cent) and severely obese (> 100 per cent), depending on the extent to which the body weight exceeds the normal weight (Stunkard 1984). In cases of severe obesity, behavioral treatment methods are unlikely to help, and surgery is indicated (Stunkard 1984).

The body mass index (BMI) is obtained by dividing weight in kilograms by height in meters squared $[W(kg)/H(m)^2]$. This index has a very high correlation with body fat (as estimated from body density), particularly when age is taken into account (Simopoulos 1986). In terms of this index, overweight is defined as a BMI of 25–30 kg/m². A BMI above 30 kg/m² constitutes obesity (Bray 1986).

Estimates of the prevalence of obesity within a given society will vary according to the criteria used. If life insurance criteria of relative weight are applied to the data from the US National Health Examination Survey for 1960–62, 15 per cent of American men aged 30–60 and 20 per cent of American women in this age range had relative weights at least 35 per cent above the desirable weight (Van Itallie 1979).

Obesity and health

The association between obesity and increases in the risk of morbidity and mortality has been well documented (e.g. Van Itallie 1979; Bray 1986). Evidence has come from studies conducted by life insurance companies (Society of Actuaries 1960; Society of Actuaries and Association of Life Insurance Medical Directors

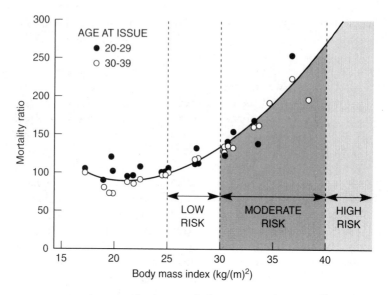

Figure 4.4   Relation of body mass index to excessive mortality
Source: Bray (1986)

of America 1979) and longitudinal studies such as the Framingham Study (Dawber 1980), the Gothenburg Study (Larsson *et al.*
1981) and the American Cancer Society Study (Lew and Garfinkel
1979).

The findings of the mortality investigations of insurance companies have been remarkably consistent over more than 75 years
(Van Itallie 1979). Figure 4.4 shows the relationship between excess
mortality and deviations in body weight observed in the most
recent of the life insurance studies, the Build Study of 1979 (Society of Actuaries and Association of Life Insurance Medical Directors of America 1979). The overall mortality rate (i.e. the ratio
of the deaths to the total population of insured lives) was taken
as 100. Figure 4.4 indicates that the minimum death rate occurred
for a BMI of 20, which is slightly less than the average weight for
the entire population. Mortality risk increased with increasing body
weight. The causes of excess death associated with overweight are
diabetes mellitus, digestive diseases, hypertension and cardiovascular diseases. There is also evidence that the distribution of the
health risk associated with obesity is affected by the distribution
of body fat. In particular, the male type of obesity, with fat stored

in the abdominal region rather than in the thighs, hips and buttocks (female obesity), seems to be associated with a greater risk to health (Krotkiewski *et al.* 1983).

If obesity increases the risk of morbidity and mortality, then losing weight should decrease these risks. Data from the life insurance industry seem to support this assumption. Thus, in individuals who had initially received substandard insurance because they were overweight but who had subsequently lost weight, life-expectancy improved to that of insured people with standard risk (Bray 1986). It has also been shown that weight reduction leads to changes in various health risk factors, including reductions in cholesterol (Thompson *et al.* 1979) and large decreases in blood pressure (Craighead *et al.* 1981; Tuck *et al.* 1981; Wadden and Stunkard 1986).

Theories of obesity

Theories of obesity can be divided into two groups: those that focus mainly on the physiological factors of weight regulation (e.g. set-point theory, fat cells), and those that emphasize psychological causes of overeating (e.g. externality, restrained eating).

Set-point theory

The notion of regulation according to a set point is familiar from the thermostats used in central heating systems, refrigerators and air conditioning systems. If one adjusts the thermostat of one's central heating system to a given temperature, the system will switch on whenever the sensors register that the temperature has dropped considerably below this set point. While it is plausible that body temperature is regulated according to a set point, the fact that there is such a wide variation in body weight seems to rule out such regulation. However, even though there is wide interpersonal variability, the body weight of most adults remains remarkably stable over time. Keesey (1986) suggested that different people may have different set points, and that for some their biological weight is set far above culture's ideal.

The most important derivation of set-point theory is that the organism will defend its body weight against pressure to change. This would certainly explain why most obese individuals have such trouble in achieving and maintaining a normal weight. There is some evidence from animals as well as humans that is consistent with set-point theory. Thus, laboratory animals adjust food intake and physical activity to compensate for starvation or forced feeding (e.g. Brooks *et al.* 1946; Adoph 1947).

Adult humans seem to respond similarly to weight displacement. Thus, during the Second World War, a group of conscientious objectors was maintained on a starvation diet for several months (Keys *et al.* 1950). Their body weight fell at first, but eventually stabilized at 75 per cent of the previous values. This equilibrium was reached partly by a decrease in basal metabolic rate and partly by a comparable decrease in the amount of metabolically active tissue. Furthermore, most returned to their previous weight once food restrictions had been removed. Similarly, when Vermont prisoners agreed to a considerable increase in their daily caloric intake, they achieved weight gains of 15–25 per cent during the half-year period. However, when the experiment terminated, these subjects soon returned to their normal weight (Sims and Horton 1968). It would seem from this evidence that some obese individuals may be fighting a battle against relentless biological forces. As Keesey (1980: 163) stated:

> If we view such [obese] individuals as different not in how they regulate body weight but rather in terms of the set-point each is prepared to defend, we might better understand why most of us remain at essentially the same body weight without so much as trying, while others remain obese no matter how hard they try to change.

Can the set point be changed? There has been a great deal of speculation but no definite evidence on this question. Among the suggested methods for resetting the set point have been lesions in the hypothalamus, exercise, extended diets and anorectic drugs (Keesey 1986).

Fat cells

The work of Björntorp, Sjöström and collaborators at the University of Gothenburg in Sweden suggested that fat cells may play an important role in the regulation of body weight (e.g. Sjöstrom 1980; Björntorp 1986). Adipose tissue (i.e. fat) is an important determinant of body weight. Weight gain can occur either through enlargement of existing fat cells (hypertrophy) or by increases in the number of fat cells (hyperplasia).

This work stimulated the popular view that the number of fat cells is determined in early childhood and that persons with adult onset of obesity are likely to have a normal number of fat cells along with enlarged cell size (Hirsch and Knittle 1970). However, Sjöström (1980) cited more recent evidence that hyperplasia can also occur in adulthood. Unfortunately, such cell multiplication cannot be undone. Björntorp *et al.* (1975) and Bosello *et al.* (1980) presented empirical evidence that dieting reduced the size of fat cells but not their numbers. Weight loss ceased when fat cell size reached a normal level. Thus, as Brownell (1982: 823) argued, "Fat cell size may set the biological limit to weight loss, whereas fat cell number may determine the weight at which this limit occurs". This could account for the poor results of dietary treatment of severe obesity. Conclusions must, however, remain tentative, because this finding was not replicated in a study by Strain *et al.* (1984).

In some ways, the implications of the work of Björntorp (1986) and Sjöström (1980) on fat cells are less encouraging than those of set-point theory. Even though set-point theory offers little comfort to the obese, it at least suggests that adults of normal weight can eat with impunity. Although the latter might gain some pounds from time to time, they are unlikely to become obese. According to research on fat cells, however, adults can increase not only the size but also the number of their fat cells, and even worse the increase in numbers is irrevocable.

Consistent with these physiological theories of obesity, evidence from twin and adoption studies suggests that weight is strongly influenced by genetic factors. Three recent studies of monozygotic twins reared apart reviewed by Bouchard and Pérusse (1993) suggested a heritability of BMI in the range 40–70 per cent, which is similar to the range of heritability estimates reported for intelligence. Bouchard and Pérusse (1993) also reported heritability estimates based on the measurement of the BMI obtained in a Norwegian sample of approximately 75,000 individuals. These data, which were used to compute familial correlations in a large number of first- and second-degree relatives, suggested a heritability of 40 per cent for BMI.

In contrast to these studies – which allowed for a substantial influence of environmental factors on body weight – recent adoption studies in which BMI data were available for both the biological as well as the adoptive relatives of the adoptees reported that the effect of the shared family environment on BMI was negligible (see Bouchard and Pérusse 1993). For example, a study of 540 adult Danish adoptees who varied across all weight categories even found the weight of the adoptees showed a strong relation to that of their biological parents but no relation to that of their adopted parents (Stunkard *et al.* 1986). However, as Bouchard and Pérusse (1993) argued, findings such as these are at odds with the strong within-family correlations observed for major determinants of body fat, such as energy intake and energy expenditure.

The externality hypothesis

This formulation was developed in the late 1960s by Schachter and his colleagues (Goldman *et al.* 1968; Nisbett 1968; Schachter and Gross 1968). Stunkard and Koch (1964) had earlier found that gastric contractions and reported hunger were highly correlated in subjects of normal weight but not in obese subjects. Schachter *et al.* therefore suggested that obese people differ from normal weight individuals in the cues that trigger their eating behavior. They argued that normal weight individuals respond mainly to internal factors – that is, to the visceral and physiological states that vary with food deprivation, such as gastric motility and blood sugar concentration. Eating behavior in overweight individuals, on the other hand, was said to be strongly influenced by external factors, such as the sight and smell of food, social stimuli and habit. Despite the plausibility of this "externality hypothesis", numerous studies failed to demonstrate these effects (for a review, see Rodin 1981). It is now widely accepted that across all weight groups there is only a weak relationship between the degree of overweight and the degree of internal or external responsiveness (Nisbett 1972; Rodin *et al.* 1977).

Dietary restraint

The construct of dietary restraint and the hypotheses relating it to eating patterns were originally developed to account for differences in the eating patterns of normal weight and obese people that had been suggested by the externality theory. Herman, Polivy and their collaborators argued (1) that obese people frequently tried to diet in an attempt to conform to social prescriptions regarding body weight, and (2) that it was the conscious restraint of eating that was responsible for the relationship between external-ity and obesity (e.g. Herman and Mack 1975; Herman and Polivy 1975). When restrained individuals force themselves to ignore or override internal demands in their attempt to diet, an insensitivity to internal hunger cues and an over-reliance on external cues is likely to develop.

More recently, Herman and Polivy (1984) incorporated their hypotheses regarding restraint into a "boundary model" of the regulation of eating. They proposed that biological pressures work to maintain food intake within a certain range. The aversive quali-ties of hunger keep consumption above a minimum level and the aversive qualities of satiety keep it below some maximum. Be-tween these two zones, there is a zone of biological indifference, where eating is regulated by non-physiological, social and environ-mental influences. Because restrained eaters frequently disregard physiological states in their attempts to diet, their range of indif-ference is wider than that of non-dieters. Restrained eaters also differ from normal people in that they have a third boundary, the "diet boundary", which is deliberately interposed between the hunger and the satiety boundaries. The diet boundary represents the restrained eater's attempt to inhibit eating before normal sa-tiety processes are activated. Once restrained eaters transgress the diet boundary, they eat until they reach the zone of satiety. Be-cause restrained eaters need more food than normal eaters to reach the dietary boundary, overeating will ensue.

Factors that interfere with cognitive control can disturb the regulation of food intake in restrained but not in normal eaters. Thus, emotional distress (e.g. Baucom and Aiken 1981; Herman et al. 1987; Schotte et al. 1990; Heatherton et al. 1991) and alcohol (Polivy and Herman 1976) have been found to disinhibit restrained eaters. A second set of factors which disturbs dietary restraint is actual or perceived dietary violation. Restrained eaters seem to perceive dieting in an all-or-nothing fashion and respond to violation with thoughts such as "I failed anyway, I might as well continue to eat". These thoughts induce them to abandon their diet for the time being (Ruderman 1986).

The effects of dietary violation on the subsequent eating behavior of restrained and normal eaters have been examined by inducing subjects to "preload" with some rich (and therefore normally forbidden) food at the beginning of what was apparently a food-tasting experiment (e.g. Herman and Mack 1975; Hibscher and Herman 1977; Knight and Boland 1989). In the first study on the effects of preload by Herman and Mack (1975), female subjects of normal weight were asked to taste ice-creams after having been given either no preload or a preload of one or two milkshakes. The subjects were divided into high restrained and non-restrained eaters on the basis of a short questionnaire, the Restraint Scale (Herman and Polivy 1975). It was expected that non-restrained eaters would eat less ice-cream after a large rather than no preload, and that restrained eaters would "binge" once they realized that their calorie intake already exceeded their daily ration. Consistent with these expectations, the intake of unrestrained subjects varied inversely with preload size, whereas that of restrained subjects showed a direct relationship. This phenomenon was assumed to result from the disruption of the cognitive control restrained eaters usually exerted over their food intake, and was called "counter-regulation".

Similar disruption was observed when subjects' knowledge of the caloric content of the preload was manipulated. For example, restrained subjects who were told they had received a high-calorie, rich pudding ate much more food at a subsequent tasting experiment than subjects who were told that they had eaten a low-calorie, diet pudding (Polivy 1976).

With the development of the boundary model, Herman and Polivy (1984) shifted the focus of their interest from obesity to anorexia nervosa and bulimia. These two eating disorders mainly afflict girls and young women. They are less common than obesity, but are, unlike the latter, considered to be psychiatric disorders. The two conditions are apparently related. They will be considered briefly here.

Anorexia nervosa is marked by self-starvation resulting from an extreme loss of weight, which in turn can lead to severe health problems. An arbitrary but useful guide for the diagnosis of anorexia is the maintenance of body weight 15 per cent below that expected for age and height (DSM-III-R; American Psychiatric Association 1987). Like anorexia, *bulimia* is also characterized by a persistent overconcern with body shape and weight. In fact, bulimia was first investigated as a symptom of anorexia nervosa, researchers dividing anorexic patients into groups of "fasters" and "bingers". The essential features of bulimia are recurrent episodes of binge eating – that is, the rapid consumption of large quantities of food in discrete periods of time, usually inconspicuously or secretly, followed by purgative behavior (e.g. self-induced vomiting; use of laxatives or diuretics). Weight fluctuations are common in bulemic persons. Most are within the normal weight range, but a few are over- or underweight.

In terms of the boundary model, anorexic patients have a very stringent diet boundary, which is often set close to the hunger boundary. The small amounts that anorexics eat are thus severely limited by this cognitive diet boundary, one that restricting anorexics seldom violate. Bulimics also have a very stringent diet boundary which, if it were consistently maintained, would make them indistinguishable from anorexics. Of course, bulimics do not always succeed in honoring the diet boundary. Binges arise from either actual or perceived transgressions of the diet boundary. This phenomenon is assumed analogous to the preload effect. A second and perhaps more frequent cause of binges is the elimination of the boundary by emotional agitation (Polivy and Herman 1987).

Even though the development of the boundary model has improved our understanding of the psychological processes involved in the patterns of disordered eating such as binge eating, the account of disordered eating offered by the boundary model is descriptive rather than explanatory. As Ruderman (1986) observed, the boundary model neither offers an explanation for the development of the various eating disorders, nor does it explain why bingers regularly violate the satiety boundary and anorexics the hunger boundary. A more comprehensive theory that integrates assumptions from set-point theory into the boundary model would be a useful development.

Conclusions

The early work on externality by Schachter and his colleagues promised to lead to a psychological theory of obesity. However, more recent findings suggest that externality may merely be a side-effect of individual battles against the physiological mechanisms of weight regulation. Research by Herman and his colleagues suggests that externality results from the conscious attempt to restrain one's calorie intake. However, even though restrained eaters are likely to be more frequent among obese rather than normal weight individuals, there is some evidence that counter-regulation may be most typical of normal weight restrained eaters (Ruderman and

Christensen 1983; Ruderman 1986). Thus, the boundary model does not offer an alternative to physiological theories of over-weight and obesity.

Treatment of obesity

Behavioral approaches
The basic assumption underlying the behavioral treatment of obesity is that overweight is due to excess food consumption (Wilson 1978; Brownell and Wadden 1986). Overeating persists for two reasons: (1) eating has immediate positive consequences, whereas the negative consequences (e.g. obesity, heart diseases) are delayed; (2) obese individuals also engage in a "faulty" eating style which contributes to overeating – they are assumed to eat more quickly and to take larger and fewer bites, sips and chews than normal weight individuals (Ferster et al. 1962; Stuart and Davis 1972).

This formulation has led to treatment strategies which have attempted to alter the energy balance by achieving a reduction in the quantity of food eaten. Three strategies have been used: (1) modification of the antecedents of eating (e.g. alteration of the environment such that high caloric food is unavailable); (2) modification of "faulty" eating styles (e.g. eating more slowly, taking smaller bites); and (3) modification of the consequences of eating (e.g. by applying immediate aversive consequences for excessive eating or by self-reinforcing abstention).

These techniques still form the backbone of most behavioral weight loss programs. To modify the antecedents of eating, the participants in such therapy programs are taught to "shop from a list", "prepare lunch after eating breakfast and dinner after lunch (to avoid nibbling)", "do not eat while drinking coffee or alcohol", "do nothing while eating", "eat only at specified times", etc. (Bellack 1977). Faulty eating habits are changed by teaching participants to "eat slowly", "take small bites", "put eating utensils (or food item) down while chewing", "take one helping at a time", "use small cups and plates", "leave some food on plate at end of meal" (Bellack 1977: 11). These strategies are still widely used, even though the assumption that obese individuals employ a "faulty" eating style has not been supported empirically (for reviews, see Striegel-Moore and Rodin 1986; Brownell 1983) and changes in eating style have been found to be unrelated to therapy success (Jeffery *et al.* 1978; Rosenthal and Marx 1978).

Because attempts to modify the consequences of overeating by aversive conditioning were not very successful, more recent programs have used financial contingencies and self-reinforcement (for a review, see Bellack 1977). With *financial contingencies*, participants are typically required to deposit a sum of money with the therapist before treatment begins. This money is then returned at weekly meetings contingent on the participant fulfilling a preset criterion (e.g. loss of a given amount of weight). The application of *self-reinforcement* relies on *self-monitoring*. Participants have to monitor and record their weight or their calorie intake. They will reward themselves when they have reached a given criterion (e.g. lost a given amount of weight or kept to a set daily calorie input). Both financial reward and self-reinforcement presuppose some kind of *goal-setting*. A recent trend has been to incorporate these behavioral techniques into more comprehensive programs that also include exercise, cognitive change and social support (Brownell and Wadden 1986; Wadden and Bell 1990).

In a survey of data from controlled trials of behavior therapy conducted in the 1970s and 1980s, Wadden and Bell (1990) concluded that the average weight loss for participants in such programs was 8.4 kg in 1985–87, compared with 3.9 kg in therapy programs conducted before 1974 (Table 4.3). This difference does not appear to be due to the greater effectiveness of more recent programs (i.e. at 0.5 kg per week, the average weight loss per week has remained the same), but to an increase in the average length of these programs.

In defence of the new programs, Brownell and Wadden (1986) argue that there is no guarantee that earlier programs would have sustained the same weight loss per week if treatment duration was increased. Furthermore, the cognitive techniques incorporated into the new programs may be helpful in preventing relapse and thus may be more relevant in later stages of treatment. This assumption is supported by the fact that the average weight loss at follow-up has improved from 4.0 kg in 1974 to 5.3 kg in 1985–87, despite the fact that follow-ups now are more than three times as long as they were in 1974. However, whereas a weight loss of 5.3 kg is substantial for somebody who is slightly overweight, it is quite insufficient for really obese individuals who may have to shed 20 kg or more.

Table 4.3 Summary of data from controlled trials of behavior therapy for weight loss

	1974	1978	1984	1985–87
Number of studies included	15	17	15	13
Sample size	53.1	54.0	71.3	71.6
Initial weight (kg)	73.4	87.3	88.7	87.2
Initial percentage overweight	49.4	48.6	48.1	56.2
Length of treatment (weeks)	8.4	10.5	13.2	15.6
Weight loss (kg)	3.8	4.2	6.9	8.4
Loss per week (kg)	0.5	0.4	0.5	0.5
Attrition (%)	11.4	12.9	10.6	13.8
Length of follow-up (weeks)	15.5	30.3	58.4	48.3
Loss at follow-up (kg)	4.0	4.1	4.4	5.3

Source: Wadden and Bell (1990).

Pharmacotherapy

Before the widespread acceptance of behavior therapy, appetite-suppressant (anorectic) drugs were the most popular treatment for obesity. These drugs were widely used because they led to substantial and effortless weight loss. Nevertheless, this type of pharmacotherapy had two major disadvantages: (1) some of the drugs (especially the amphetamines) were likely to be abused, and (2) the weight loss achieved with drug therapy could rarely be maintained.

Anorectic drugs have now become much safer. Pharmacotherapy would therefore be useful in cases of severe obesity, if the problem of the maintenance of weight loss could be solved. Because the maintenance of drug-induced weight loss requires some change in lifestyle, the combination of anorectic drugs with behavior therapy would seem to constitute an optimal therapy. The use of drugs would achieve a fast and effortless weight loss, while the techniques of behavior therapy would lead to the required changes in lifestyle.

To test this hypothesis, Craighead *et al.* (1981) compared the combined effects of drug and behavior therapy with the impact of drug or behavior therapy used alone (Figure 4.5). Although those subjects who received pharmacotherapy (fenfluramine) alone or in combination with behavior therapy had significantly greater weight losses than those on behavior therapy alone (14.5 and 15.3 kg *vs*

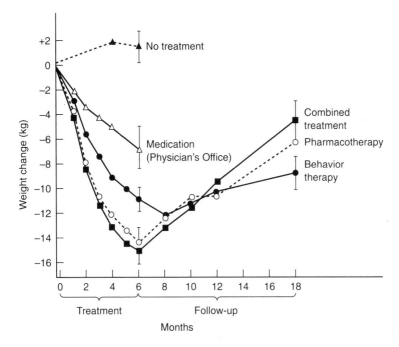

Figure 4.5 Weight change during 6 months of treatment and 1 year follow-up (from Craighead *et al.* 1981).

10.9 kg), a 1 year follow-up showed a striking reversal in the relative efficacy of treatments. The behavior therapy patients regained significantly less weight (1.9 kg) than the subjects in the pharmacotherapy (8.2 kg) or the combined treatment conditions (10.7 kg). The resulting trend in net weight loss now favored the behavior therapy alone condition (net loss of 9.0 kg) over the other two conditions (net loss pharmacotherapy alone 6.3 kg; net loss combined treatment 4.6 kg). Thus, somewhat surprisingly, therapy was not only ineffective in helping to maintain the weight losses due to pharmacotherapy, but the long-term effects of behavior therapy were actually poorer if patients had also received pharmacotherapy than if they had not.

It is interesting to speculate how the addition of medication could compromise the effectiveness of behavior therapy (though note a failure to replicate by Craighead 1984). It seems possible that the reduction in appetite caused by the anorectic drug prevented individuals from learning the behavioral techniques in the presence of competing hunger cues. Thus, when the drug was stopped, they might have been unprepared to cope with the resulting increase in hunger. However, this interpretation was not supported by findings of a second study conducted by Craighead (1984), in which she used pharmacotherapy either during the first or during the second half of a 16 week behavior therapy program. The long-term results of these two sequences were no different from those of a combined treatment in which medication was administered for the total 16 weeks of behavior therapy.

A second interpretation could be derived from theories of cognitive control, such as Bandura's (1986) notion of *perceived efficacy*. Patients who received the combined treatment may have attributed their weight loss to medication and may thus have failed to develop the feeling of control over their weight that is important for the maintenance of weight loss. The validity of this explanation could have been tested if Craighead and colleagues had included a condition in their studies that combined placebo medication with behavior therapy. However, even though some doubt may remain about the theoretical interpretation of these results, the practical implications are obvious – the long-term effects of behavior therapy are not improved by pharmacotherapy.

Very low-calorie diets

Although total fasting results in significant weight loss, much of the weight loss consists of lean body tissue as well as body fat. This protein malnutrition could have serious consequences for hepatic, renal and pulmonary functions (Blackburn *et al.* 1986). Very low-calorie diets are supplemented fasts that are designed to spare lean body mass through the provision of 70–100 grams of protein a day in a total of 300–600 calories. Very low calorie diets produce average weight losses of 20 kg in 12 weeks (Blackburn *et al.* 1986). They appear to be safe when undertaken under careful medical supervision and limited to periods of 3 months or less. As with drug treatment, the major problem with very low-calorie diets is the rapid regain in weight after the termination of treatment.

Fortunately, in this case, the combination of a very low-calorie diet and behavior therapy proves to be quite effective. In a study by Wadden *et al.* (1983), patients were treated for 6 months with a program of a very low-calorie diet and behavior modification designed specifically for weight loss maintenance. The subjects lost an average of 20.5 kg during treatment, of which they regained only 2.1 kg at 1 year follow-up.

These results were replicated by Wadden and Stunkard (1986) in a more controlled study, in which subjects were randomly assigned to a very low-calorie diet, behavior therapy or a very low-calorie diet plus behavior therapy (combined treatment). The subjects in the diet condition were treated for 4 months in a program that included 2 months of a very low-calorie diet and 2 months of a diet of 1000 calories. The subjects in the behavior therapy condition were given a 6 month course of behavior therapy. The combined treatment incorporated the diet into this 6 month program. At the end of the treatment, the subjects in the diet group had lost 14.1 kg, those in the behavior therapy group 14.3 kg and those in the combined treatment group 19.32 kg.

At 1 year follow-up, the diet group had regained 9.5 kg, compared with 4.8 kg in the behavior therapy group and 6.4 kg in the combined treatment group. Thus, the diet group had the lowest net loss with only 4.6 kg lost, the behavior therapy group had an intermediate loss of 9.5 kg, and the combined treatment group had the highest loss of 12.9 kg. The loss experienced by the combined treatment group replicates the results of Wadden *et al.* (1983), and thus demonstrates that this combination of behavior therapy and a very low-calorie diet reliably produces clinically significant weight losses.

Exercise

Most of the weight reduction techniques described earlier aim at the input side of the energy equation. However, because overweight individuals consume more energy than they expend, increasing energy expenditure would offer an alternative or additional means of reduction. The neglect of exercise, particularly in the early weight control programs, had been justified by the belief that exercise does not use up many calories (e.g. 2 miles of walking uses only about 200 calories), and that this minor effect is likely to be outweighed by the increase in appetite resulting from such exercise.

In contrast, studies that examined the impact of exercise alone and in combination with behavioral techniques have found increases in exercise to result in substantial weight loss. For example, Dahlkoetter *et al.* (1979) assigned subjects randomly to one of

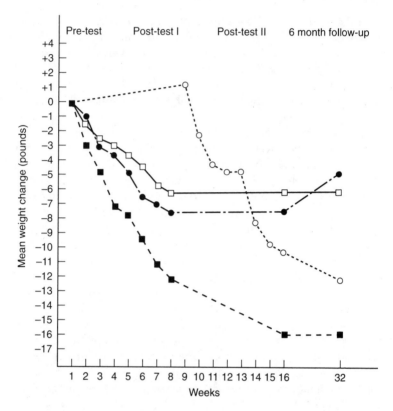

Figure 4.6   Weight change for groups receiving treatment for eating habits (□), exercise treatment (●), combination of these treatments (■) and controls (○)
Source: Dahlkoetter *et al.* (1979)

four groups: (1) exercise, (2) eating habits (3) combination, and (4) delay-of-treatment control group. Each group met for eight 1 hour sessions. The exercise group focused primarily on energy expenditure methods of weight reduction; the eating habit group was taught behavioral techniques of dietary control; the combination group received a package of both treatments; the delay-of-treatment group also received the combined treatment but only after an 8 week wait. The results after the first 8 weeks (post-test 1) indicated significant improvements for all treatment groups in comparison with the control group (see Figure 4.6). The combination group showed the greatest improvement in weight and body circumference. At 8 week follow-up (post-test 11), only the combination group had continued to lose weight. Once treated, the delay-of-treatment control group showed a weight loss similar to that of the combination group. Studies by Duddleston and Bennion (1970), Harris and Hallbauer (1973) and Stalonas *et al.* (1978) also found that exercise in combination with diet or behavioral management produced greater weight loss than did single exercise, dietary or behavioral intervention. It is particularly impressive that the effects of exercise were often stronger at the follow-up than immediately after the termination of treatment (Harris and Hallbauer 1973; Stalonas *et al.* 1978; Dahlkoetter *et al.* 1979).

Because there is no indication that drop-out rates are higher under conditions that combine exercise and dietary intervention, the greater weight loss in the combined treatment groups does not seem to be due to a self-selection in terms of motivation. And yet the impact of exercise on weight is difficult to explain through physiological processes, because exercise uses up relatively few calories. To resolve this inconsistency, researchers have suggested that exercise results in an increase in metabolic rate that outlasts the actual duration of the exercise and that this increase in metabolic rate is sufficient to counter the lowering of the metabolic rate caused by dietary restriction (Thompson *et al.* 1982).

In view of the difficulties involved in identifying the physiological mechanisms that mediate the impact of exercise on weight, it might be more fruitful to speculate about a psychological interpretation. In our earlier discussion of the negative impact of anorectic medication on the maintenance of weight loss, we suggested that the patients who received the combined treatment may have attributed their weight loss to medication and may thus have failed to develop the feeling of control over their weight that is necessary to maintain weight loss. Similarly, one could argue that adherence to an exercise regimen increases people's feelings of self-efficacy. Such an increase in the sense of self-efficacy and the feeling of control over their weight might have led the exercise group to be more motivated in following the dietary instruction. This interpretation would also explain the finding that the impact of exercise on weight was even stronger at long-term follow-up.

Findings that exercise improves the effectiveness of behavioral programs of weight reduction suggest that these programs should incorporate exercise regimens as part of the intervention. Furthermore, including exercise has the additional advantage that it increases coronary fitness and decreases the loss of lean tissue. Whereas weight loss through diet alone is approximately 75 per cent fat and 25 per cent lean tissue, the combination of exercise and diet reduces the loss of lean tissue to approximately 5 per cent (Brownell 1982). Recent comprehensive programs for managing obesity therefore include exercise as an integral part of treatment (Brownell and Wadden 1986).

Self-help and self-help groups

It is plausible that, before going to a therapist, individuals who are overweight and want to lose weight will try one of the many popular weight-loss diets. In Schachter's (1982) study described earlier, of 40 people who had made active attempts to lose weight, 62.5 per cent had achieved normal weight and a further 10 per cent, though still overweight, had lost substantial amounts of weight. The people interviewed by Rzewnicki and Forgays (1987) in a replication of Schachter's study were somewhat less successful in losing weight.

If we follow Schachter's logic, self-help programs by organizations such as TOPS (Take Off Pounds Sensibly), who offer classes throughout the USA and several other countries, should largely draw on those individuals who have failed to cure themselves. The key element of TOPS is weekly meetings to provide group support, with weigh-ins constituting the high point of these meetings (Stunkard 1986). Assessment of the effectiveness of this program is difficult because of the high drop-out rate. An early cross-sectional study of TOPS by Stunkard et al. 1970) revealed that the membership then was almost exclusively female, white and middle class. The average member was a 42-year-old woman whose ideal weight was 54.0 kg and who had entered TOPS weighing 82.0 kg. She stayed in TOPS for 16.5 months and lost 6.8 kg. A later longitudinal study showed that by failing to take account of the high drop-out rate, these earlier figures considerably overestimated the effectiveness of TOPS (Garb et al. 1974). According to Stunkard (1986), in one study nearly 67 per cent of members dropped out during the first year and these were persons who had been least successful at losing weight.

Commercial weight-loss organizations such as Weight Watchers have added three important elements to the programs pioneered by non-profit groups such as TOPS: behavior modification, inspirational lectures drawn from successful members, and a carefully designed nutritional program (Stunkard 1986). But they also suffer from the problem of attrition. Two prospective studies of a representative sample of the members of a large commercial organization found that approximately half the members dropped out during the first 6 weeks (Volkmar *et al.* 1981).

That the effectiveness of self-help groups can be improved is suggested by a study conducted in Norway (Grimsmo *et al.* 1981). In Norway, self-help organizations for weight control have grown into a nationwide movement with 80,000 people participating. They work in small groups (8–12 members), meeting once a week for 8 weeks, monitoring body weight each time. Members are given dietary information, and are encouraged to do physical exercise and give up alcohol. The fee has to be paid in advance and the drop-out rate is less than 10 per cent.

In a first study, 33 female members were monitored throughout the course and then interviewed 3, 6 and 12 months later. At the end of the course, their average weight loss was 6.5 kg. Twelve months later, they had regained on average 1.0 kg. Thus with a net loss of 5.5 kg, these women were doing better than the average individual undergoing behavior therapy.

In a second prospective study, the authors obtained data from the "slim-club hostesses" on initial weight, weight at weekly intervals, and end results of 11,410 individuals who participated in a course during the spring of 1977. The average weight loss of the 10,650 participants (93.3 per cent) who completed the course was 6.9 kg (with drop-outs included, it was still 6.4 kg). Even though these data were collected by the slim-club hostesses, the fact that they agreed with those obtained in the earlier study and that members could monitor how hostesses filled in their charts, increases one's trust in these findings. In a retrospective survey of the long-term effects of this self-help program, the authors found that the average weight remained stable for the first 2 years but then began to rise. After 5 years, participants had regained half of their initial weight loss. These findings and the data reported by Schachter (1982) tend to indicate that at least for mild cases of obesity, the help of professional therapists may not be essential.

Conclusions

Obesity is an important medical problem that is related to an increase in the risk of serious diseases such as diabetes and hypertension and to increased mortality. Despite popular beliefs that obesity is caused by overeating, the evidence on differences in the food intake of obese and normal weight individuals is not very conclusive. Physiological theories such as set-point theory suggest that the weight of obese individuals is set at a higher point and that therefore they might be fighting a battle against relentless biological forces when attempting to gain their ideal weight. This set point may in part be determined by the number of an individual's fat cells.

Fortunately, there have been great advances in the development of comprehensive treatment programs in recent years. Even though the substantial weight losses achieved by pharmacotherapy or very low-calorie diets alone seem to be difficult to maintain, the combination of very low-calorie diets (but not pharmacotherapy) with behavior therapy has led to weight losses that are clinically significant and have been maintained over extended periods after treatment. Thus, statements made only a few years ago that people are more likely to recover from most forms of cancer than from obesity (Brownell 1982) may have been overly pessimistic.

Summary and conclusions

This chapter has presented evidence on the impact of smoking, alcohol abuse and excessive eating on health. Without doubt, the findings on health deterioration are strongest for cigarette smoking, which has been identified as the single most important source of preventable mortality and morbidity in each of the reports of the US Surgeon General produced since 1964. Although the empirical evidence on the health impact of *moderate* alcohol consumption is more ambiguous, there can be no doubt that *alcohol abuse* is also a very serious public health problem which impairs social and occupational functioning in addition to health. Finally, obesity is linked to increases in the risk of serious diseases such as diabetes and hypertension and to increased mortality.

Once people smoke, drink too much alcohol or have a weight problem, these appetitive behaviors are difficult to change. Even though therapy might help individuals to act on their intentions to adopt more healthy habits, the strength of their intentions may be at least as important as the therapy for the eventual outcome. Because of the difficulties in changing these health-impairing habits, we argue that primary prevention is a more effective health strategy than behavior change. We further suggest that programs of primary prevention should not only rely on persuasion and health education but also on planned changes in the rewards and costs associated with these health behaviors. These latter strategies may be less applicable for weight control. However, there is evidence that cigarette consumption and alcohol abuse can be influenced by increases in the tax on tobacco and alcohol products, by instituting stricter age limits or by a reduction of availability through limiting sales.

Suggestions for further reading

Blane, H.T. and Leonard, K.E. (Eds) (1987). *Psychological theories of drinking and alcoholism*. New York: Guilford Press. An authoritative overview of a wide range of psychological theories as they relate to drinking problems and alcoholism.

Brownell, K.D. and J.P. Foreyt (Eds) (1987). *Handbook of eating disorders*. New York: Basic Books. A collection of chapters by leading authorities in the field on causes, health impact and treatment of obesity.

Hurley, J. and Horowitz, J. (Eds) (1990). *Alcohol and health*. New York: Hemisphere. Written by leading authorities in the field of alcoholism, the chapters in this edited book provide a comprehensive discussion of the epidemiology, health effects and treatment of alcoholism.

Leventhal, H. and Cleary, P.D. (1980). The smoking problem: A review of the research and theory in behavioral risk modification. *Psychological Bulletin*, 88, 370–405. A very thoughtful discussion and review of studies concerned with the initiation, maintenance and therapy of cigarette smoking in children and adults.

5 / BEHAVIOR AND HEALTH: SELF-PROTECTION

In this chapter, we focus on health-enhancing or self-protective behaviors, such as eating a healthy diet, exercising, avoiding behaviors that are essential to the transmission of AIDS (unprotected sex, needle sharing) and protecting oneself against accidental injuries. The division of health behaviors into excessive appetites and self-protection is somewhat arbitrary. However, there is some difference between these two types of behavior with regard to the extent to which they are under volitional control. While people frequently need therapy to enable them to stop smoking, to give up alcohol or to lose weight, it would be rather unusual if people required therapy to reduce the salt content of their food, take up jogging, to practice safe sex or to fasten their seatbelts.

Healthy diet

Obesity is not the only health risk that is related to diet. There is growing evidence that important ingredients of our diet, when taken in excess, may have a deleterious effect on our health. Thus, a high intake of salt (sodium chloride) has been related to the development of hypertension and ultimately cardiovascular disease (Frost *et al.* 1991; Law *et al.* 1991a, 1991b), and excessive fat consumption has been linked to an elevated morbidity and mortality from atherosclerotic heart disease and even cancer (Weinstein and Stason 1985; Greenwald *et al.* 1986).

Salt intake and hypertension

Hypertension is a major risk factor for strokes and coronary heart disease. There may be many causes of hypertension, but the factor that is most frequently cited is intake of salt. Although the role of salt remains controversial, the World Health Organization (WHO) Expert Committee on Prevention of Coronary Heart Disease felt sufficiently confident of the link to advocate a reduction in the amount of salt consumed (WHO 1982). Since then, a group of British researchers has published a comprehensive meta-analysis of most of the published studies on the relationship between salt intake and blood pressure (Frost *et al.* 1991; Law *et al.* 1991a, 1991b). Their analysis tends to justify the recommendation given by the WHO experts.

This meta-analysis was based on data from three types of studies: (1) *between-population* studies that related the average blood pressure of different populations to average sodium intake; (2) *within-population* studies that related individuals' blood pressure to salt intake; and (3) *intervention* studies that tested whether a reduction in salt intake resulted in a reduction in blood pressure. It could be demonstrated not only that the relationship was significant in all three types of study, but also that it was similar across the different data sets.

Law *et al.* (1991b) concluded from these findings that a modest reduction in daily salt intake by 2–3 grams would result in a modest fall in blood pressure after a few weeks. Other researchers have argued that a reduction in salt intake is only beneficial for *some* individuals, namely those who are particularly salt-sensitive, because of a decreased capacity of the kidney to excrete sodium (e.g. Haddy 1991). However, since a moderate reduction in salt intake is essentially without side-effects, it should be tried first as a therapy for patients with mild-to-moderate hypertension. Even if drug therapy is finally required to lower blood pressure, dietary sodium restriction may reduce the effective dose of the drug and thus also reduce its side-effects (Haddy 1991).

Cholesterol and coronary heart disease

Of all the dietary risk factors, the relation between excessive fat consumption and coronary heart disease has been studied most extensively. The hypothesis specifying the role of dietary cholesterol in the development of coronary heart disease has been modified over the years with the emergence of new empirical evidence. This has indicated that there are good and bad fats, just as there are good and bad cholesterols. In its most recent form, the hypothesis states that excessive ingestion of saturated fat leads to an elevation of low-density lipoproteins (LDL-cholesterol) in (blood) serum; this causes atherosclerosis, which in turn brings about clinical manifestations of coronary heart disease (Stallones 1983).

Food fats can be divided into two categories – vegetable and animal fats. The latter may be further divided into three subcategories – dairy fats, land animal fats and marine fats, including the fats of fish and of marine mammals such as whales or seals. The properties of the fatty acid composition of these types of food fats are very different. Vegetable and marine fats are unsaturated and contain substantial amounts of polyunsaturated fatty acids, mainly linoleic acid. Dairy and meat fats are much more saturated and contain only small amounts of linoleic acid (Turpeinen 1979).

Cholesterol is a fat-like substance. Contained in most tissues, it is also the main component of deposits in the lining of arteries. Serum cholesterol has been classified into high- and low-density lipoproteins (Avogaro 1984). Elevated serum cholesterol and low-density lipoproteins are assumed to be positively associated with the prevalence of coronary heart disease. Since these specifications of the hypothesis have only been made during the last few decades, most of the data that are available on serum cholesterol or on food fats cannot be related to these distinctions. Thus, in most population-based research, dietary fat has to be used as an index of saturated fat and serum cholesterol as an index of serum levels of low-density lipoproteins (Stallones 1983).

Large epidemiological studies have shown significant positive correlations between cholesterol levels in the blood and the incidence of coronary heart disease (e.g. Kannel *et al.* 1971; Dawber 1980). There is now wide consensus that, in industrial societies, the risk of coronary heart disease rises as serum cholesterol increases over most of the serum cholesterol range (Stallones 1983).

There is much less consensus, however, regarding whether serum cholesterol levels are really caused by dietary factors. While some authors (e.g. Lefebvre 1986) believe that diet has a direct impact on serum cholesterol levels, others (e.g. Kaplan 1984, 1988) argue that serum cholesterol levels are mainly determined by genetic factors. Proponents of the dietary viewpoint stress that population studies comparing dietary habits and serum cholesterol across groups with diverse eating habits have generally found a strong relationship between dietary cholesterol and serum cholesterol (Blackburn 1983). For example, the so-called "Seven Country Study" (Keys 1980), which was carried out in the USA, Japan and five European countries, found a very high correlation between the ingestion of saturated fats and serum cholesterol levels ($r = 0.89$) and between the fat content of the diet and the incidence of coronary heart disease ($r = 0.84$).

Supporters of the genetic perspective (e.g. Kaplan 1984, 1986) point out that epidemiological research has consistently failed to demonstrate a relationship between dietary cholesterol and serum cholesterol *within* a given culture. For example, 24 hour dietary recall interviews were conducted with a sample of approximately 2000 men and women residents in the community of Tecumseh (Michigan, USA) to determine the influence of diet on serum cholesterol levels. Trained interviewers obtained detailed descriptions of all foods consumed during 24 hours before venipuncture for lipid determination. No relationship could be found between dietary variables and levels of serum cholesterol concentration for men or women. Similarly, in the Evans County, Georgia study, 25 white males were selected whose serum cholesterol values were very low (160 mg/dl or less) and compared with 26 who had very high values (260 mg/dl or more). These two groups did not differ significantly in any of the dietary variables assessed (Stulb *et al.* 1965).

There is also little evidence of a relationship between diet and coronary heart disease from these studies. Stallones (1983), who reviewed six US epidemiologic studies and one British study in which dietary assessment was done at the beginning of a period of observation, reported that individuals who subsequently developed coronary heart disease either differed not at all in their total caloric and fat consumption patterns from the persons who remained well or they differed in the direction opposite to that predicted by the hypothesis (see Figure 5.1). Findings from population-based studies of genetic factors further support the genetic argument. In general, these studies find support for a sizeable genetic influence and little indication of environmental factors (for a review, see Segal *et al.* 1982).

Some support for the dietary hypothesis comes from prospective studies of the effects of dietary interventions. For example, Turpeinen (1979) reported that marked changes in diets among

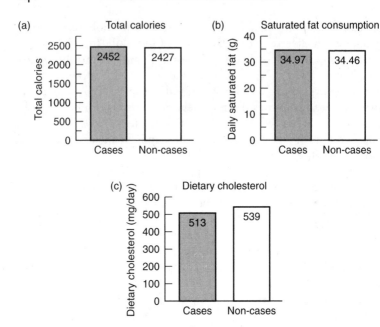

Figure 5.1   Dietary factors and mortality due to heart disease:
Differences in consumption for adults who survived or died. (a) Based
on 914 cases and 21,713 non-cases; (b) based on 544 cases and
16,123 non-cases; (c) based on 752 cases and 21,389 non-cases
Source: Kaplan (1985)

men in two Finnish mental hospitals were associated with a statistically significant decline in mortality from coronary heart disease in that population. A number of other studies have reported
similarly positive results for coronary heart disease (for a review,
see Holme 1990). However, even though the reduction in dietary
cholesterol appears to have resulted in a reduction in mortality
from heart disease in most intervention studies, mortality averaged
over *all causes* was not affected by experimental dietary intervention. Reductions in coronary deaths were associated with increases
in deaths from other causes (for a review, see Jacobs 1993). Similarly, a controlled trial using pharmacotherapy demonstrated that
pharmacologic reduction of serum cholesterol in hypercholestero-
lemic individuals (individuals with high levels of serum cholesterol)
also resulted in a considerable decrease in the risk of mortality
from coronary heart disease (Lipid Research Clinics Program 1984a,

1984b). Again, there was no significant overall reduction in mortality from all causes.

It is difficult to draw conclusions on the basis of the available evidence. There is little doubt that high levels of serum cholesterol are related to the development of atherosclerosis and increase the risk of coronary heart disease. There is also some evidence to suggest that dietary factors play a role in high serum cholesterol levels. However, the reduction of elevated serum cholesterol through diet or drugs does not reduce overall mortality.

Exercise

If one were to conduct a survey of beliefs about what people should do to improve their health, regular exercise would probably be mentioned by most respondents. Thus, a majority of healthy American adults in 1973 and 1978 agreed with the statement "Exercise is important for good health" (Oldridge 1984). However, such beliefs do not always translate into action. Even in the USA, where health consciousness appears to be much higher than in Europe, only 15 per cent of the population exercise regularly and intensively enough in their leisure time to meet current guidelines for fitness (Oldridge 1984).

Nevertheless, there is strong evidence that regular vigorous dynamic exercise decreases the risk of hypertension, coronary heart disease and mortality from all causes. Such *aerobic* exercises, intended to increase oxygen consumption, include jogging, cycling and swimming. All of these are marked by their high intensity, long duration and need for high endurance. The regimen most effective in developing and maintaining cardiorespiratory fitness is to exercise 3–5 days a week for 15–60 minutes per session at more than 60 per cent of maximum heart rate (American College of Sports Medicine 1979). This exercise prescription is designed to expend a certain amount of energy per session. Thus, an hour of walking or a 20–30 minute run would use between 250 and 300 kilocalories (kcal) for a person weighing 70–80 kg (Oldridge 1984).

Exercise and physical health

Some of the pioneering research on the health benefits of vigorous physical activity was conducted by Morris and his colleagues in the UK, who related both vocational and leisure time physical activity to a reduction in the risk of coronary heart disease (e.g. Morris *et al.* 1953, 1980b). Even though these early studies suffered from a number of methodological weaknesses, their findings have since been widely replicated (for reviews, see Powell *et al.* 1987; Paffenbarger and Hyde 1988).

Occupational activity

Paffenbarger and his colleagues at Stanford University continued the work of Morris on the impact of occupational activity on health (Paffenbarger and Hale 1975; Brand *et al.* 1979). In their long-term study, a group of 3975 longshoremen (i.e. wharf laborers who load and unload cargo) aged 35–75 years were followed for a 22 year period from 1951 to 1973. Apparently, their work activity involved a wide range of energy expenditure which was evaluated by physical measurements taken in actual on-the-job situations and then converted into energy-output values (kcal/week).

It was found that 11 per cent (n = 395) of the longshoremen died of coronary heart disease during the 22 year period. Men who expended 8500 or more kcal/week at work (heavy work) had significantly less risk of fatal heart disease at any age than those men whose jobs required less energy. The relative risk of individuals engaged in moderate and light physical activity was nearly twice that of workers doing the heavy jobs. There was practically no difference in risk between individuals engaged in moderate or light physical activity. The negative relationship between physical activity and coronary mortality remained when other known factors that contribute to coronary heart disease, such as heavy cigarette smoking and high systolic blood pressure, were controlled for. Similar findings were reported in other studies relating work activity to mortality from coronary heart disease (for a review, see Powell *et al.* 1987). While most of these studies used all-male samples, some studies have replicated the negative relationship for both sexes (e.g. Brunner *et al.* 1974; Salonen *et al.* 1982).

As the researchers themselves are the first to admit, "a leap of faith is required in any non-experimental study when we attempt to draw causal interpretations from statistical associations" (Brand *et al.* 1979: 60). One weakness of these kinds of correlational studies is that it is nearly impossible to control for the possibility that symptoms of clinical illness several years previously may have led to switches from higher to lower energy output jobs. Thus workers who became ill while in a high-activity job may have been switched to one involving lower activity before their death. However, this interpretation is rendered less plausible by the fact that Brand and his colleagues were able to rule out the possibility that job changes less than 4.5 years prior to death accounted for the relationship between work activity and coronary health.

Leisure time activity
It would be very difficult for people who work in sedentary jobs to achieve, in their leisure time, such a high level of energy expenditure as the longshoremen in the study described above. Fortunately, much lower levels of leisure time energy expenditure appear to be sufficient to achieve a marked decrease in the risk of coronary heart disease. This was first demonstrated by Morris and his colleagues, who reported that middle-aged male office workers who kept fit and engaged in vigorous sports during an initial survey in 1968–70 had an incidence of coronary heart disease in the next $8\frac{1}{2}$ years that was somewhat less than half that of their colleagues who undertook no vigorous exercise (Morris *et al.* 1980a).

These findings were replicated in the USA with a large sample of former male students of Harvard University (Paffenbarger *et al.* 1978, 1986). In this study, 16,936 male alumni who had entered Harvard between 1916 and 1950 returned a questionnaire concerning their physical activities (e.g. walking, stair climbing, sports) either in 1962 or in 1966. A second questionnaire in 1972 identified the non-fatal heart attacks that had occurred in the meantime. Records of fatal heart attacks were obtained for a period of 12–16 years.

During the first 6–10 years, there were 572 first heart attacks. Age-specific rates of coronary heart disease declined consistently with increasing energy expended per week on exercise. Energy expenditure was again aggregated into a composite index of physical activity and expressed in terms of kilocalories per week. Men with an index below 2000 kcal/week were at 64 per cent higher risk than classmates with a higher index. Risk of heart attack was clearly related to present-day activity, rather than to activity during student days. Thus, the fact that an alumni had engaged in competitive sports as a student was unrelated to risk of heart attack in later life. Furthermore, as Figure 5.2 indicates, the inverse relationship between activity and risk of heart attack could be demonstrated

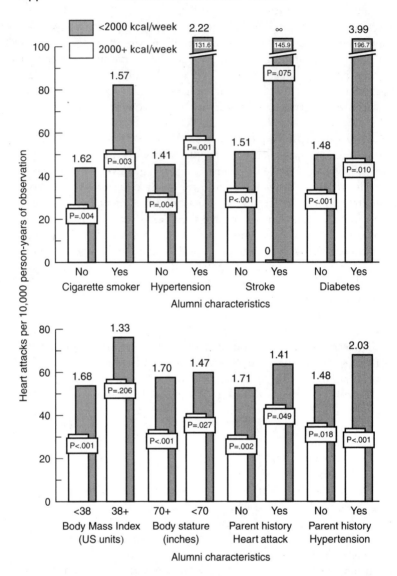

Figure 5.2 Physical activity and first heart attack (from Paffenbarger *et al.* 1978). *Note*: Given here are paired combinations of the physical activity index and other characteristics of Harvard male alumni. Relative risk is calculated as follows:

$$\frac{\text{rates for alumni with low physical activity index}}{\text{rates for alumni with high physical activity index}}$$

even when other risk factors were controlled for. This is very important, since risk factors such as body weight or smoking are strongly and negatively related to exercise adherence.

Of the alumni who returned the questionnaire, 1413 died during the 12–16 years of follow-up. Exercise was negatively related to mortality. Death rates from coronary heart disease as well as from all causes declined steadily as energy expenditure increased from less than 500 to 3500 kcal/week. Beyond this point, there was only a slight increase in rates. Men who expended less than 2000 kcal/week were at 31 per cent higher risk of death than more active men.

Physical fitness

In most of the studies reviewed here, some screening was used to exclude individuals who already suffered from some diagnosed illness. However, the most extensive clinical screening was probably done in a study by Blair et al. (1989), in which male and female participants received a preventive medical examination at a clinic at the outset of the study. All individuals who had a personal history of heart attack, hypertension, stroke or diabetes were excluded, as were subjects who had abnormal responses to a resting or exercise electrocardiograph.

Physical fitness, which can be considered an objective indicator of habitual physical exercise, was measured directly by a treadmill exercise test. The average follow-up of the participants (10,224 men and 3120 women) was slightly more than 8 years. Fitness was negatively related to mortality. This inverse relationship was significant for mortality from all causes and for mortality from coronary heart disease. It remained significant even after statistical adjustment for age, smoking habits, cholesterol level, systolic blood pressure, fasting glucose level and parental history of coronary heart disease.

Control of confounding variables

Since none of the studies on the impact of exercise used random assignment of subjects to levels of physical activity, the issue of temporal priority (i.e. whether the assumed cause really preceded the assumed effect) is difficult to establish. When individuals are free to determine their own level of physical activity, it is likely that they choose to become less active with the onset of some disease process. Health screening of participants at the beginning of a study enables exclusion of individuals who already suffer from coronary heart disease or some other serious illness. However, with medical diagnoses being less than perfectly reliable, even careful medical screening could not rule out the possibility that the lowering of activity levels was due to some undiagnosed illness. However, as Powell and co-workers (1987) argued, if self-selection by illness were an important factor, studies with medical screening before the observation period should show smaller and less consistent associations between activity and health than those without prior screening. In their extensive review of studies on physical activity and coronary heart disease, Powell *et al.* (1987) failed to find evidence for such a difference.

A second strategy to safeguard against self-selection by illness is to omit all deaths or illnesses that occurred during the first 2–3 years of follow-up after exercise assessment. This was done in the Harvard alumni study (Paffenbarger *et al.* 1986) and in the study relating physical fitness to all causes of mortality (Blair *et al.* 1989). A strong negative relationship still pertained between exercise and death from cardiovascular disease. Since one would expect the strength of the inverse relationship to weaken considerably over time if individuals with subclinical heart disease were over-represented in the inactive group, the persistence of a strong relationship makes an interpretation in terms of this type of self-selection less plausible.

There is a second type of self-selection, however, that cannot be controlled by these procedures – namely, self-selection by risk factors. There is evidence that people who are older, of lower socioeconomic status, overweight or smokers are more likely to drop out of voluntary exercise programs than younger, middle- or upper-class, normal weight, non-smoking individuals (for a review, see pp. 151–3). Since all of these variables are also related to an increased risk of morbidity and mortality, this type of selection could account for the health difference. However, in many of the studies reported earlier (e.g. Paffenbarger *et al.* 1978, 1986; Blair *et al.* 1989), the health benefit of exercise could be demonstrated even when these risk factors were statistically controlled.

In conclusion, the evidence from these and other studies on the health impact of physical exercise is quite consistent in demonstrating an inverse relationship between physical activity and coronary heart disease. Even though a controlled intervention study is still needed in this area, the studies reported earlier have been very thorough in controlling for all suspected confounding variables.

Studies of leisure time activity have suggested that a weekly energy expenditure in excess of 1500–2000 kcal is sufficient to reduce the risk of mortality from heart disease. It is left to the reader to judge whether one can, as most writers in this area appear to do, consider a vigorous half-hour run daily or an hour of walking a moderate level of physical activity that is attainable by most adults. Fortunately, for those who are satisfied with less than maximal health benefits, the relationship between activity level and health appears to be monotonic, at least for leisure time activity.

Mediating processes

A number of biological mechanisms have been proposed to explain how physical activity might prevent the development of coronary heart disease (Powell *et al.* 1987). It has been suggested that muscular activity may directly protect the cardiovascular system by stimulating the development of collateral vessels that support the heart muscle. There is evidence from animal studies that physical activity increases the diameter of epicardial coronary arteries (e.g. Kramsch *et al.* 1981) and enhances coronary collateral development (Neil and Oxendine 1979). However, there is no evidence from human studies to support this hypothesis (Powell *et al.* 1987).

Exercise could also prevent sudden cardiac death by enhancing myocardial electrical stability. This could have been responsible for the lower rate of sudden deaths reported for the more active subjects in several studies. There is some evidence that physical training increases cardiac parasympathetic tone in humans (Kenney 1985). Parasympathetic stimulation reduces ventricular fibrillation that can be caused by insufficient blood supply to the heart muscle (Kent *et al.* 1973). There is also evidence from animal studies of a heightened resistance to ventricular fibrillation after exercise training (e.g. Billman *et al.* 1984).

Finally, physical exercise may have beneficial effects on factors that contribute to the development of coronary heart disease, such as being overweight and high blood pressure. Evidence has shown that exercise has positive effects on weight control (Thompson *et al.* 1982), and it also appears to reduce the risk of hypertension (Paffenbarger *et al.* 1983). However, since the positive effects of exercise on health have been demonstrated in studies that controlled for weight and hypertension (e.g. Paffenbarger *et al.* 1978), these factors are unlikely to be the major mediators of the exercise–health relationship.

Exercise and psychological health

It is widely believed that aerobic exercise has a beneficial effect on mental health. Aerobic fitness programs such as jogging, dancing or swimming have come to be frequent prescriptions for treating depression (McDonald and Hodgdon 1991). Although most reviews of the empirical research on the impact of regular exercise on mental health (e.g. Folkins and Sime 1981; Morgan and O'Connor 1988) have concluded that the causal nature of this relationship is rather unclear, a recent meta-analysis of 90 studies that appeared before 1989 drew more definitive conclusions regarding the impact of aerobic exercise on a variety of psychological states (McDonald and Hodgdon 1991).

The impact on mood

Mood is usually defined as an individual's feelings at a specific moment and thus reflects a temporary state rather than an enduring trait. From a meta-analytic review of 26 correlational and experimental studies that have been conducted on the impact of exercise on mood, McDonald and Hodgdon (1991) concluded that aerobic fitness training produces positive changes in mood states. However, findings from a recent experimental study by King et al. (1989), which was not included in the meta-analysis, suggest that, at least in healthy populations, the immediate impact of regular exercise may be limited to those psychological variables which are closely associated with exercise-induced physical changes, such as satisfaction with shape, appearance and fitness. It is possible, however, that the changes in satisfaction with these aspects may in turn have a significant impact on other psychological variables.

Exercise and depression

McDonald and Hodgdon (1991) concluded on the basis of a meta-analytic review of 15 studies that aerobic exercise had a positive impact on depressive symptomatology and that this impact was greatest for subjects who were initially depressed. Findings from studies by McCann and Holmes (1984) and Doyne et al. (1987) illustrate the beneficial effect of aerobic exercise on depressive symptomatology.

The subjects in the McCann and Holmes study were 43 female students who had scored above the cut-off point for mild depression on the Beck Depression Inventory (BDI). These individuals

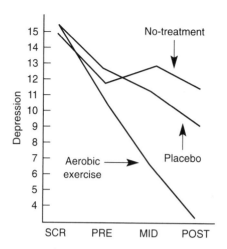

Figure 5.3 Depression and exercise (from McCann and Holmes 1984). *Note*: Given here are mean screening (SCR), pre-treatment (PRE), mid-treatment (MID) and post-treatment (POST) depression scores for subjects in aerobic exercise, placebo and no-treatment conditions

were randomly assigned to either an aerobic exercise treatment condition in which they participated in vigorous exercise for 1 hour twice a week for 10 weeks, a placebo treatment condition in which they practiced relaxation training, or a no-treatment condition. Depression was assessed with a self-report measure (BDI) before, during and after the intervention period. The results indicated that subjects in the exercise condition showed a greater reduction in depressive symptomatology than did subjects in the other two conditions. Furthermore, the impact of the exercise was most marked after 5 weeks. Continuing the exercise for another 5 weeks did not substantially add to the effect (see Figure 5.3).

These findings were replicated by Doyne *et al.* (1987) in a study of 40 women who had been screened for major or minor depressive disorder. These women were randomly assigned to an 8 week running, weightlifting or non-exercise control condition. The subjects were also assessed before, during and after the treatment by various self-rating scales of depression, which included the BDI. The results indicated statistically and clinically significant decreases in depression in both the exercise groups relative to the control group. These improvements were remarkably consistent across the different measures and were reasonably well maintained at 1 year follow-up.

Mediating processes

A number of physiological and psychosocial mechanisms have been suggested to account for the impact of exercise on depression (for a review, see Morgan and O'Connor 1988). It has been suggested that aerobic exercise may facilitate the production of brain norepinephrine (Beckman et al. 1979). Low norepinephrine levels in the central nervous system have been suspected as a cause of some depressions. Another hypothesis has been that improved mood state following exercise is stimulated by the release of endorphins, which are opoids produced by the body (Steinberg and Sykes 1985).

At a more psychological level, it has been argued that exercise may reduce anxiety and depression because it distracts individuals and prevents them from focusing on their problems (Bahrke and Morgan 1978). However, while this could account for some immediate effects of exercise on anxiety and mood, it is difficult to see how it could explain long-term effects.

A better explanation of such long-term effects is the assumption that exercise may increase individual feelings of self-efficacy. The fact that one is regularly exercising or even participating in an exercise group may increase one's feeling of being disciplined, effective and competent. Some of the positive effects of exercise may also stem from factors associated with exercise, such as social activity and a feeling of involvement with others. Thus, for example, cycling with friends, swimming with a companion, or running with others may improve mood because of the companionship involved.

The determinants of regular exercise

Who are the people who keep fit and how can we persuade those who do not to engage in regular exercise? Research on the attitudes which characterize participants in exercise programs has often relied on rather global measures of attitudes toward physical activity and sports such as the Physical Estimation and Attraction Scales (Sonstroem 1978; Sonstroem and Kampper 1980). These global measures have been only moderately successful as predictors of recruitment into exercise programs (for reviews, see Dishman

1982; Oldridge 1984; Sonstroem 1988). This is not surprising, since, as we discussed in Chapter 2, global attitudes are notoriously poor predictors of specific behaviors.

According to the compatibility principle discussed earlier (Chapter 2), the best predictor of the performance of specific exercises should be the individual attitude and intention toward performing this exercise. Riddle (1980) collected data on attitudes and behavioral intentions toward regular jogging from several hundred joggers and non-exercisers using a mailed questionnaire that was based on the theory of reasoned action (Fishbein and Ajzen 1975). In support of this model, the intention to jog was successfully predicted from the attitudinal and normative components of the model and the correlation between intention and behavior was high.

Riddle (1980) also found a number of meaningful differences between the beliefs of joggers and non-exercisers. Non-exercisers thought jogging would require too much discipline, take too much time and make them too tired. Joggers were more likely than non-exercisers to believe that regular jogging would have positive effects, and they also evaluated being in good physical and mental condition more positively. Non-exercisers also indicated that it was unlikely that important reference persons (particularly their physicians) thought that they should jog regularly.

A prospective study conducted by Valois et al. (1988) found somewhat lower, but still significant relationships between attitudes, intentions and behavior. These authors assessed specific attitudes, norms and intentions to predict self-reported physical activity measured 3 weeks later. One interesting result of this study was that the prediction of behavior from behavioral intention could be significantly improved when a measure of past performance of physical activities was entered into the regression analysis. Since past behavior is likely to reflect behavioral control, this finding suggests that the theory of planned behavior, an extension of the theory of reasoned action which includes a perceived behavioral control component, might have been more successful in predicting exercise behavior.

According to the theories of reasoned action and planned behavior, program adherence should be predicted from attitudes toward *continued participation* in a program of physical activity, rather than from attitudes toward the specific physical activity. Since only individuals with positive attitudes toward physical activity are likely to be recruited into the group of exercisers, program adherence should only be weakly related to general attitudes toward physical exercise. In line with this argument, global measures of attitudes toward physical activity have typically been unsuccessful in predicting adherence, even in cases where they were reasonable predictors of recruitment into the exercise program (e.g. Sonstroem and Kampper 1980).

In contrast, studies that assessed attitudes and behavioral intentions toward continued program participation were fairly successful in predicting program adherence (e.g. Olson and Zanna 1982; Jonas et al. 1993). For example, in a prospective study of a sample of more than 100 men and women who had registered in university fitness courses at the University of Tübingen (Germany) for a 4 month exercise program, Jonas et al. (1993) predicted the intention to participate ($R^2 = 0.55$) and actual program participation ($R^2 = 0.13$) on the basis of subjects' attitudes toward continued participation, perceived social norms and perceived behavioral control. Olson and Zanna (1982) predicted attendance at a fitness center from assessments of behavioral intentions, perceived social norms and attitudes toward exercising and adherence.

Unfortunately, from a perspective of health education, many of the other variables that have been found to be related to exercise participation and adherence, such as age, education, smoking and proximity to the exercise facility, are less open to influence (Dishman 1982; Oldridge 1984; Sonstroem 1988). Even self-motivation, which has been found to be significantly related to adherence in several studies (Dishman and Gettman 1980; Dishman et al. 1980; Dishman and Ickes 1981; Olson and Zanna 1982), appears to be a fairly stable personality disposition. Self-motivation is conceptualized as a behavioral tendency to persevere independent of situational reinforcements and is measured by a paper-and-pencil test.

Of the physical variables, body fat and body weight appear to be major determinants of adherence to exercise programs. Thus, in one prospective study, Dishman and Gettman (1980) found that body fat, body weight and self-motivation (which were determined at the beginning of the study) predicted 45 per cent of the variance in adherence of a sample that consisted of 21 male cardiac patients and 45 healthy male individuals. More than half of this variance (24 per cent) was accounted for by percent body fat.

What conclusions are we to draw about how to persuade people to exercise and how to increase adherence to exercise programs?

Researchers in this area seem to agree that people join exercise programs to obtain some health-related benefits (e.g. improvement in cardiovascular fitness, weight-loss), but the fact that they stay because the program is convenient and enjoyable suggests a two-step procedure. However, little is yet known about the features that make exercise programs enjoyable.

Since convenience is likely to be a predictor of involvement as well as adherence, mass media campaigns should not only emphasize the health-related benefits of specific exercise, but they should also point out that it takes less effort to stay healthy than most people might anticipate. Furthermore, whereas it is difficult to persuade people to join a health club or even to take a daily half-hour walk, it may be much easier to persuade them to rearrange their daily lives and become more physically active.

That individuals can be persuaded to change minor routines has been demonstrated by Brownell et al. (1980). These authors observed that only 6 per cent of the people in shopping malls, train and bus stations tended to use stairs rather than elevators. When a simple sign pointing out the benefits of exercise was placed at the bottom of the stairs and escalators, stair use was nearly tripled. Similarly, one might be able to persuade people to walk or cycle to work instead of driving (which would also be good for environmental reasons) or, at least, to park one's car further away from one's place of work. Who knows, people who enjoy these small activities and who have become more physically fit as a result may even decide to take up jogging or join an exercise class.

The primary prevention of AIDS

In 1991, more than 800,000 people worldwide were suffering from the acquired immune deficiency syndrome (AIDS) according to an estimate by WHO. This is only the tip of the iceberg. WHO estimates that at least 30 million people could be infected with the AIDS virus by the year 2000 (*Time*, August 2, 1992). There is presently neither a cure nor a vaccine to prevent AIDS. And yet people can escape the infection by avoiding behaviors that are essential to the transmission of the AIDS virus. Thus, programs aimed at changing behavior are at present the only feasible strategy to halt the AIDS epidemic.

The cause of AIDS

AIDS is caused by a virus, called the human immunodeficiency virus (HIV), which attacks the immune system. The immune system reacts with the formation of antibodies. Although these antibodies do not play a protective role as they do in more familiar virus infections, they can be used as indicators of the presence of the virus. These antibodies can be detected in the blood serum by simple tests, 2 weeks to 3 months after infection. Individuals who have developed antibodies are said to be seropositive. But even before the development of antibodies, the individual can be infectious to others through sexual intercourse or blood donations.

The period between contracting the virus and developing the symptoms of AIDS is highly variable. Some individuals develop the symptoms quite quickly, whereas others remain free of symptoms for as long as 8–9 years. The average incubation interval is now thought to be 7–10 years (Osborn 1989). Due to this long incubation period, there is still some disagreement about what proportion of HIV-infected individuals will finally develop AIDS. However, recent evidence reveals the prognosis to be not very favorable. Studies of long-term cohorts of seropositive patients suggest the possibility that most if not all infected persons will progress to AIDS (Curran *et al.* 1988).

Infection with HIV damages the immune system by infecting and killing one type of white blood cell, the T-helper cells. The T-helper cells serve an important function in the regulation of the immune system. They stimulate other cells to mount an attack on invading germs. By infecting and ultimately killing the T-helper cells, the HIV stops the process of responding to invading germs at the beginning and thus severely reduces a person's ability to fight other diseases. Without a functioning immune system to ward off other germs, the individual is vulnerable to infection by germs (bacteria, protozoa, fungi, other viruses) and malignancies, which would ordinarily not have been able to gain a foothold. Usually AIDS is diagnosed through the presence of unusual opportunistic infections (i.e. infections that use the opportunity of lowered resistance) or unusual forms of cancer (e.g. Kaposi's sarcoma, a cancer of the skin and connective tissues). The AIDS virus also appears to attack the nervous system, causing damage to the brain.

Modes of transmission

The virus is transmitted by the exchange of cell-containing bodily fluids, notably blood, semen and vaginal secretions. In the USA, most sexual transmission of HIV has occurred between homosexual men. The risk for these men is strongly associated with the number of sexual partners and the frequency with which they are the receptive partner in anal intercourse (Curran *et al.* 1988). Although insertive anal intercourse is also likely to be infectious, there is evidence that the risk of infection during intercourse is greater when the seropositive person inserts his penis into a seronegative person than vice versa. HIV can be spread by vaginal as well as anal intercourse, although infectivity is lower, probably because there is less likelihood of lesions (Hulley and Hearst 1989).

The risk of becoming infected is considerably reduced by the use of condoms. For example, gay men who used condoms only some of the time were six times more likely to become infected with HIV than those who used condoms all of the time (Detels *et al.* 1989). However, studies of AIDS infection in HIV-discordant couples suggest that condoms and spermicides are not completely safe even with vaginal sex (Hulley and Hearst 1989). In a survey of homosexual men interviewed as part of the Amsterdam cohort study who reported that they used condoms, condoms were reported to have slid off or become torn during anogenital sex in 3.7 per cent of cases (de Wit *et al.* 1993b). When failure rates were calculated in relation to the type of lubricant, condoms used with water-based lubricants failed less frequently (1.7 per cent) than condoms used with no lubricants (5.9 per cent) or with oil-based lubricants (10.3 per cent).

Among intravenous drug users, the risk of infection is not caused by the drug use *per se*, but by the sharing of injection equipment. The HIV is carried in contaminated blood left in the needle or syringe and the virus is injected into the new victim when dirty syringes or needles are re-used. In general, the risk of contracting AIDS through contact with infected blood is very high. Thus, blood transfusions from infected donors carry an extremely high risk of infection (Friedland and Klein 1987).

Fortunately, there is no evidence that HIV can be transmitted through casual contact. It does not seem to enter the body across skin that is intact, and thus is not transmitted by touching, hand shaking, sharing eating utensils, sneezing or living in the same household (Curran *et al.* 1988). Thus, in studies of households where one person was HIV-infected, none of over 400 family members was infected except for sex partners or children born to infected mothers (Curran *et al.* 1988). Even though the virus is present in saliva, the concentration is low and there is no evidence that the virus can be transmitted by kissing.

The epidemiology

The first report of AIDS in the USA involved fewer than a dozen men in the summer of 1981. Early in 1991, the number of AIDS cases reported from 159 countries had risen to 334,215 according to WHO (*Frankfurter Allgemeine Zeitung*, March 9, 1991). Sixteen per cent of these cases came from the USA, 6 per cent from Europe and 69 per cent from Africa. Since not all countries report their cases and since these reports are often outdated, WHO estimated that the actual number of individuals suffering from AIDS was more like 800,000 (*Frankfurter Allgemeine Zeitung*, March 9, 1991). Due to the mode of transmission, AIDS mainly affects a younger segment of the population.

Until now, the highest risk groups in the USA and Europe have been homosexual/bisexual men and intravenous drug users. In the USA, 92 per cent of the AIDS patients are male. The category of homosexual/bisexual men account for just over 70 per cent of the total if one includes the 8 per cent who are intravenous drug users. Intravenous drug use is the sole risk factor for 17 per cent of AIDS patients. When the overlap with homosexual or bisexual men is noted, as much as 25 per cent of the epidemic could be due to drug-related behavior (Osborn 1989). However, recent reports suggest that the importance of heterosexual transmission of AIDS is increasing. Heterosexual patients without any other risk factor comprise the fastest growing group of AIDS cases in the USA (Jacobs 1993).

Prior to the institution of protective measures to make the blood supply secure, hemophiliacs and other blood recipients could contract AIDS through blood transfusions. Thus, by the end of 1987, 2 per cent of the adults and 12 per cent of the children with AIDS in the USA were believed to have acquired the disease in this manner (Friedland and Klein 1987). Although only 1 per cent of the adults with AIDS have hemophilia, 70–80 per cent of persons with hemophilia have already acquired HIV. It is estimated that

12,000 persons in the USA were infected with HIV through trans-fusions before the screening of donated blood and plasma for antibody to HIV began in 1985 (Friedman and Klein 1987).

As in the USA, the incidence of AIDS in Northern Europe is highest among homosexual and bisexual men. In Spain and Italy, however, the majority of cases are intravenous drug users. In Central Africa, HIV transmission is linked to the re-use of scarce needles, and a lack of infection control procedures in hospitals and clinics. It is also clearly related to heterosexual rather than homosexual intercourse (Batchelor 1988). Thus, in many African countries, the rate of AIDS is roughly equal for both sexes.

Due to the long incubation period between infection and the development of symptoms, the number of AIDS cases represents only a small proportion of the individuals infected with HIV. According to the US Centers for Disease Control (1987), the number of HIV-infected individuals in the USA is estimated to be between 1 and 1.5 million (5–10 million worldwide). However, while only 1989 AIDS cases were reported in the USA in 1981, this number climbed to 43,339 (17.2 per 100,000 population) in 1991 (Aral 1993). There are also wide regional differences. For example, from April 1991 to March 1992, the reported number of AIDS cases per 100,000 persons varied between 0.2 in North Dakota and 122.4 in the District of Columbia (Aral 1993).

Obviously, the prevalence is much higher in known risk groups. The US Centers for Disease Control (1987) summarized 140 studies of the prevalence of antibodies to HIV in homosexual men and intravenous drug users in the USA. According to this research, the prevalence of HIV is in the order of 20–50 per cent among homosexual men. For example, the population-based Men's Health Study found a prevalence of just under 50 per cent in San Francisco (Winkelstein *et al.* 1987). The prevalence among intravenous drug users is somewhat lower (0–20 per cent), except for some north-eastern cities. In Newark and New York, the seroprevalence among intravenous drug users has reached 50–60 per cent (Hulley and Hearst 1989), compared with 10 per cent in Chicago and San Francisco (Des Jarlais *et al.* 1985; Chaisson *et al.* 1987).

Behavioral risk reduction among homosexuals

When it became known that the risk of HIV infection can be considerably reduced or even eliminated by a change in those behaviors that help to transmit the disease, the homosexual communities at the centers of the epidemic reacted with a variety of community-level intervention efforts. Even though these interventions have rarely been formally evaluated at the level of specific programs, a number of large-sample longitudinal studies were initiated in 1983 and 1985 to assess behavior change in the gay community. Many of these studies were conducted in San Francisco – for example, the San Francisco Men's Health Study (Winkelstein et al. 1987) and the San Francisco Behavior Cohort (McKusick et al. 1985a, 1985b). But there were also studies conducted in other parts of the USA (e.g. New York: Martin 1987) and in Europe (e.g. Amsterdam: van Griensven et al. 1988). These studies suggested that the knowledge of the AIDS risk resulted in substantial behavior change. Since 1990, however, evidence has begun to emerge suggesting that the practice of unsafe sexual behavior may be increasing again in some of these samples (e.g. Ekstrand and Coates 1990; de Wit et al. 1992).

The San Francisco Men's Health Study investigated a cohort of more than 600 homosexual men (Winkelstein et al. 1987). These were selected in 1984 from the 19 San Francisco census tracts with the highest cumulative incidence of AIDS using multistage household probability sampling and face-to-face interviews. The participation rate was 59 per cent. Information from a biannual assessment conducted between 1984 and 1986 revealed a 60 per cent reduction in receptive and a 66 per cent reduction in insertive unprotected anal intercourse. There was also a substantial decline in the average number of sexual partners during this period. The fact that the proportion of men who were seropositive at the beginning of the study showed hardly any increase during this period provides evidence that the reduction in risk behavior resulted in a stabilization of the prevalence of HIV infections in this sample.

Similar levels of risk reduction were also reported from other studies, such as the San Francisco Behavior Cohort Study, a questionnaire study of more than 600 homosexual men recruited from bars, from bathhouses and through advertisements (McKusick et al. 1985a; Coates et al. 1989), and a study of a New York City sample of more than 700 self-identified gay men (Martin 1987). In these studies, the proportion of men who reported unprotected anal intercourse in the late 1980s was typically less than 20 per cent.

However, the evidence from San Francisco and New York, both epicenters of the epidemic, may lead one to overestimate the extent of the behavior change that occurred in the gay communities as a result of the AIDS epidemic. Studies conducted in less affected areas typically reported higher levels of high-risk behavior among homosexual men, even though substantial reductions in risk behavior had occurred (for a review, see Catania *et al.* 1989). For example, in the Amsterdam Cohort Study, a longitudinal study of more than 600 homosexual men who were repeatedly questioned about their sexual behavior between 1984 and 1988, 46 per cent reported giving up unprotected anogenital sex, but nearly 30 per cent still regularly practiced unprotected anal intercourse, and a further 19 per cent engaged in unprotected anal intercourse some of the time (de Wit *et al.* 1992).

Furthermore, after years in which substantial reductions could be observed in the practice of unsafe sex, several studies have recently reported evidence for a reversal of these trends (e.g. Ekstrand and Coates 1990; de Wit *et al.* 1992). For example, in the Amsterdam Cohort Study, the proportion of men who reported engaging in unprotected anogenital sex during the previous 6 months increased from a low of 29 per cent in the first 6 months of 1991 to 41 per cent in the second half of the same year. Most of this change was due to an increase in the number of men who practiced unprotected anal intercourse with casual partners from 13 to 24 per cent (de Wit *et al.* 1993a).

There are a number of methodological limitations to this type of research which might have biased findings. Thus, the frequent use of samples of convenience and the large refusal rates raise troublesome questions about the representativeness of the samples and the generalizability of the findings. Not only were the majority of respondents in these studies white and well-educated (Becker and Joseph 1988), but the motivation underlying the decision to participate in such a survey is also unclear (Catania *et al.* 1990). If people refuse to participate because they practice high-risk sexual behavior and do not want to admit it, these studies might actually underestimate high-risk behavior.

Another potentially biasing factor arises from the longitudinal methodology used in these studies. Repeated assessments over time may elicit greater self-monitoring of one's sexual behavior and increased effort to change risky behavior. It seems plausible, therefore, that repeated interviews of the same individuals may produce behavior changes that would not have occurred otherwise. However, Catania *et al.* (1991) recently compared the reports of a longitudinal cohort with those of three cross-sectional samples of gay men interviewed at the same time and found similar increases in condom use across samples.

Behavioral risk reduction among intravenous drug users

Intravenous drug users are the second largest group at risk of AIDS in the USA and Northern Europe. Since the virus is not transmitted by the drug use itself but by the sharing of needles or syringes, it would seem easier to change this behavior than to influence men who are homosexual to reduce their number of sexual partners and to use condoms. However, unlike the gay community, which is relatively organized and of comparatively advantaged educational and socioeconomic status, more intravenous drug users often come from minority groups and their level of education is typically lower (Becker and Joseph 1988). Furthermore, even though the sharing of injection equipment in the pre-AIDS days was used to express social bonding within the intravenous drug-use subculture, such equipment is not freely available to intravenous drug users. There are legal restrictions on the sale of injection equipment in many states of the USA. Furthermore, pharmacists often refuse to sell syringes and needles to suspected drug users (Des Jarlais and Friedman 1988). Therefore, intravenous drug users often rent their injection equipment at locations where this is available, so-called "shooting galleries", or they use the "house works" (injection equipment kept by the dealer for customers who want to inject immediately). Needles and syringes may be rented repeatedly until they are no longer usable. Thus, sequential anonymous sharing of blood-contaminated needles and syringes occurs among large numbers of persons (Friedland and Klein 1987). As Des Jarlais and Friedman (1988) point out, the use of shooting galleries and house works breaks the limited protection that would occur if drug users shared equipment only within friendship groups.

Studies of AIDS-related behavior change among intravenous drug users suggest that many have changed their behavior in response to the AIDS threat. In many US states, mass communication concerning the AIDS threat was supported by outreach programs, in which trained former addicts were employed as educators for intravenous drug users not receiving treatment (Des Jarlais and Friedman 1988). The purpose of these programs is to educate drug addicts about AIDS, to encourage them not to share needles and to teach them methods of sterilizing injection equipment (a 10 per cent solution of household bleach and water appears to be sufficient to inactivate HIV).

Becker and Joseph (1988) and Des Jarlais and Friedman (1988) have extensively reviewed studies conducted in New York, San Francisco, Amsterdam and Edinburgh, which together indicate significant behavioral changes among intravenous drug users in order to avoid AIDS. The validity of the self-reported changes in injection behavior is supported by studies in New York City that suggest that there has been a marked increase in the demand for sterile injection equipment (Des Jarlais et al. 1985). Similarly, in the Netherlands, organized intravenous drug users established needle exchange systems in many large cities. This system allowed intravenous drug users to return used injection equipment and to exchange it for new equipment without cost. Since the AIDS threat, the needle exchange system has been greatly expanded (Des Jarlais and Friedman 1988).

Other studies have indicated that drug addicts in some cities did not change their high-risk behavior, even though they knew that sharing needles was dangerous. Des Jarlais and Friedman (1988) concluded from their review of the literature that, although information about AIDS and the transmission of AIDS is needed by intravenous drug users to generate motivation for risk reduction, this information is not sufficient. The means for either reducing drug injection or easily obtaining sterile injection equipment have to be provided in order to achieve a reduction in risk behavior. As they pointed out, the cities in which large percentages of intravenous drug users reported a behavior change were also cities in which there were increased means for behavior change (e.g. safer injections, treatment). It is important to note that there is no evidence that providing the means for safer injections increases the extent of drug injection.

Research on interventions

There have been several intervention efforts to induce people to modify their AIDS-risk behavior. However, as Fisher and Fisher

(1992) noted in their comprehensive review of these studies, few of these interventions have been stringently derived from social psychological theories of attitude and behavior change. Instead, the majority of interventions have been based on an "informal blend of logic and practical experience" (p. 463). Fisher and Fisher (1992) also argued that although providing subjects with information about the AIDS risk *and* motivating them to avoid unsafe sexual behavior is a necessary condition for behavior change, it may not be sufficient for a reduction in the risk of AIDS. In addition, certain behavioral skills, such as the ability to communicate with, and be assertive with, a potential sexual partner are necessary for practicing AIDS prevention. Individuals must be able to negotiate AIDS prevention behavior with a partner and be capable of leaving situations in which safe sex cannot be negotiated (Fisher and Fisher 1992).

That interventions including social skills training can be quite effective has been demonstrated by Kelly *et al.* (1989). The participants in their study were 104 gay men of apparently good health but at very high behavioral risk for HIV infection. These were randomly divided into an immediate intervention group and a waiting list control group. The members of the intervention group were taught – through modeling, role play and corrective feedback – how to exercise self-control in relationships and to resist coercive pressure from a sexual partner to engage in unsafe practices. Evaluation at the end of the training program indicated that the members of the intervention group significantly reduced their frequency of unprotected anal intercourse and increased their frequency of condom use. At 8 month follow-up, frequency of anal intercourse had decreased to near zero levels and condoms were used in 77 per cent of those few anal intercourse occasions that took place. Whether this kind of intervention program would be successful with teenagers, members of various minority groups or with intravenous drug users remains to be seen.

Few studies have examined the impact of communication campaigns on the reported behavior of the heterosexual population. Although heterosexual transmission has so far been of much less importance in the spreading of AIDS in the USA and Europe, it has become the fastest growing component of HIV spread (Aral 1993). It is not only intravenous drug users who provide an entry into the heterosexual population; there is also evidence for both men and women that there are substantial levels of sexual interaction across the boundaries of sexual orientation (Reinish *et al.* 1988).

The results of a survey conducted in New York before and after an advertising campaign in the city in 1987 directed at AIDS prevention in unmarried, sexually active men and women between the ages of 18 and 34, are not very encouraging. On the positive side, awareness of sexual transmission of HIV increased, and more than 80 per cent agreed that sexually active people should carry condoms and that women should tell their sexual partner to use condoms. However, the number of reported sexual contacts during the previous months had not changed, and 60 per cent failed to use a condom regularly (Fineberg 1988). This is in line with surveys among college students, which find that although students appear to be knowledgeable about HIV infections, they have not adequately adopted preventive behavior (Patrick *et al.* 1992).

Summary and conclusion

It is evident that there has been a substantial reduction in the practices that are known to be involved in the transmission of HIV. Thus, despite the lack of controlled studies, there can be little doubt that the marked behavior changes that have been documented in the research reported above have been a reaction to the diffusion of information about AIDS. However, in view of the terrible nature of the illness and the high risk involved in behaviors such as needle sharing or unprotected receptive anal intercourse, particularly in the epicenters of the epidemic, more information is needed to understand why some individuals still persist in engaging in this behavior. Such understanding could then be used to effect behavior change. Furthermore, the evidence of a recent increase in unsafe sexual practices suggests that promotion efforts for safer sexual practices among homosexual men have to be continued.

Injury prevention and control

One consequence of the dramatic change in causes of death during this century is that injuries have become the major cause of death during the first four decades of a person's life. Whereas previously the greatest threat to the health and welfare of children came from infectious diseases, inadequate nutrition and sanitation, injuries are now the cause of more deaths to children in the USA and most Western countries than the next six most frequent causes combined (Christophersen 1989). Therefore, the loss of potential years of life before age 65 due to injury death is far greater than the loss due to any of the other leading causes (Waller 1987). Thus, a decrease in the death rate due to injuries would save more person-years of life than a decrease in any of the other causes of death.

The epidemiology

In the USA, one accidental death occurs every 6 minutes (National Safety Council 1986). Approximately two-thirds of the injury deaths in the USA in 1986 were due to unintentional injuries, and one-third were due to intentional injuries (suicides, homicides). The most frequent causes of violent death were injuries sustained in motor vehicle collisions, followed by suicide, homicide, falls and deaths due to fire or flames.

Unlike deaths, which are reportable, less severe injuries are often not reported. Morbidity due to injury is therefore more difficult to assess than mortality. According to one estimate, one injury is likely to occur every 4 seconds in the USA, resulting in a weekly total of 173,100 injuries (National Safety Council 1986). At this rate, there are 8.7 million injuries per year in the USA (Christophersen 1989).

The control of injury

Injury is usually defined as bodily "damage resulting from acute exposure to physical and chemical agents" (Haddon and Baker 1981: 109). Injury occurs when these agents impinge on the body at a level which the body cannot resist. There are three public health strategies for injury control: *persuasion, legal requirements* and *structural change*. While the first two strategies rely on inducing people to change their behavior, the third approach reduces the risk of injuries by changing the design of equipment, vehicles or the environment.

Strategies of injury protection can be placed on an active–passive continuum, according to the effort they require from the person implementing that strategy. For example, the most active strategy to lower the risk that children get scalded by hot tap-water would be to prevent children from running hot water. This would involve forbidding them to approach the hot water tap and monitoring them whenever they are near any of the taps. A less active strategy would involve lowering the setting of the water heater to a level where the water is no longer scaldingly hot. This would require only one action, the adjustment of the thermostat. The least active strategy would be a legal requirement for manufacturers of water heaters to fix settings at a level that does not allow water heaters to discharge water that is scaldingly hot (Wilson and Baker 1987). This would make water heaters safe for children without any actions from their caretakers. There is consensus among experts in the area of injury control that protecting people through environmental changes or changes in vehicles or equipment used, whenever possible, is more effective than mass education or the introduction of legal requirements to induce self-protective behavior.

Persuasion

As with other areas of health behavior, it is very difficult to persuade people to take actions that protect them against accidental injuries. The use of seatbelts provides a good example. In most countries, only 10–20 per cent of drivers used their belts before the introduction of laws requiring their use, even though their use requires very little effort and they reduce mortality risk to wearers involved in accidents by 60 per cent according to some estimates (e.g. Robertson 1986). It should therefore have been easy to persuade people to use their belts.

Despite this, media campaigns persuading drivers to use seatbelts have been notoriously ineffective (Robertson 1986, 1987). In one study, radio and television advertisements urging seatbelt use were employed extensively in one community, moderately in a second and not at all in a third. In the 5 weeks of the study, no significant change in seatbelt use occurred that could be attributed to the campaign (Fleischer 1972, reported by Robertson 1987). Similarly disappointing were the results of a 9 month seatbelt use campaign on one cable of a dual-cable television system used for marketing studies. Although the advertisements were shown nearly 1000 times, often during prime-time viewing, there were no differences in seatbelt use between those households viewing the experimental cable and those viewing the control cable or the community at large at the end of the campaign (Robertson *et al.* 1974).

Why are people so resistant to persuasion, even when it is in their own self-interest to take action? One reason is that persuasive strategies usually focus on knowledge and motivation, and thus affect only two of the factors that are involved in self-protection. Obviously, knowledge of both the risk and the protective action is a prerequisite to self-protection. But even if individuals know that a certain action will protect them against some danger, they might forget to do so at the time in question. This is particularly likely to happen when the necessity for the protective behavior arises infrequently and is also not consistently related to a sequence of action.

But even if people are reminded of the self-protective action, they might not be motivated to engage in that action because it is effortful and/or because the likelihood of an accident seems remote. For example, the reminder systems installed in most US cars in the early 1970s did little to increase seatbelt use (Robertson 1987). In such cases, compliance with protection recommendations can often be increased by linking additional incentives to the behavior and/or by making the behavior less effortful. For example, if children's seats could be made to clip in more easily, or even be permanently installed to be unfolded from underneath the seat, people would probably be more likely to use them every time they have small children as passengers in their cars.

Finally, people might fail to take a self-protective action if they have insufficient control over the behavior that is required. For example, parents have only limited control over the behavior of small children. Thus, whenever the safety of small children is involved, structural changes to make the child's environment safer will be particularly effective. Similarly, people caught for drunken driving are often people with alcohol problems, who may be unable to control their drinking (Robertson 1987). In such cases, a withdrawal of their driver's license until they have overcome their alcohol problem would be more effective than education concerning the dangers of drunken driving.

Legal requirements

Legal requirements are effective to the extent that they succeed in linking new incentives to a given behavior. Thus, seatbelt laws introduce a new incentive for seatbelt use, namely, the avoidance of paying a fine. There is ample evidence for the success of legal requirements in inducing behavior change. For example, when the Swedish Government made seatbelt use compulsory for front-seat passengers in private cars, seatbelt use increased from 30 to 85 per cent within a few months (Fhanér and Hane 1979). In New York, where seatbelt use ranged from 10 to 20 per cent prior to the introduction of a seatbelt law in 1984, it increased to 45–70 per cent after the law entered into force in early 1985. The introduction of these laws also resulted in substantial reductions in the deaths of vehicle occupants (Robertson 1986).

Laws requiring parents to restrain their infants or toddlers during motor vehicle travel, which has been adopted by all US states, has also been very effective. According to observational surveys at shopping centers in 19 cities, the rate of child restraint use increased from roughly 20 per cent in 1980 to 80 per cent in 1990 (Graham 1993). Recent estimates suggest that the number of infant and toddler fatalities in motor vehicle crashes are 25–40 per cent less than they might have been if child restraint laws had not been adopted (Graham 1993). Laws requiring the use of helmets by motorcyclists were similarly successful (Robertson 1986).

For legal requirements to be effective, the behavior that is enforced has to be easily monitored. Thus, the law limiting blood-alcohol concentration in drivers is difficult to enforce. According to some early estimates, only 1 in 2000 drivers illegally impaired by alcohol is actually arrested for the offense (Robertson 1984). However, roadside sobriety checkpoints are increasingly employed to increase the probability that drunk drivers will be detected and apprehended. Furthermore, swiftness of punishment has been enhanced by new state legislation that authorizes police to suspend a driver's license before conviction on the basis of evidence that the driver has exceeded the legal blood-alcohol limit (Graham 1993).

Even though laws offer additional incentives to encourage self-protective behavior, they still have to rely on the motivation of the individuals at risk to be effective. This also limits their usefulness. Thus, they often have least impact on those subgroups that are at greatest risk, because those likely to be most reckless are least likely to comply with legal requirements. For example, seatbelt laws seem to be least observed by the young and the alcohol-impaired (Robertson 1978).

Structural changes
The great advantage of the structural approach to injury control which changes the environment to make it safer is that it protects

people without requiring any effort on their part. An example of a successful structural change was the introduction of smaller containers for children's aspirin. The number of children dying after the ingestion of bottles of flavored aspirin decreased substantially after bottle sizes were reduced to contain only sublethal doses, even when all the tablets in a bottle were consumed. This strategy was more effective than the introduction of childproof caps that had to be replaced after every use and that some children were able to circumvent (Wilson and Baker 1987).

In the area of traffic safety, the introduction of federal standards in the USA in 1968 that required new cars to meet performance criteria for crashworthiness and crash avoidance resulted in an estimated reduction of 14,000 traffic deaths per year by 1982 (Robertson 1986). Substantial further reductions in traffic fatalities will be achieved once all cars are equipped with air bags that inflate automatically in the more severe frontal crashes. It has been estimated that this will reduce traffic fatalities in the USA by 9000 deaths per year (Robertson 1986).

Conclusions

The opinion of experts in the area of injury control that passive strategies are preferable to active strategies is compelling, since any active strategy for controlling injury depends on convincing a large number of people to change their behavior in a way that protects them against injury, which has proved very difficult to do. Persuasion is particularly liable to fail when the behavior is effortful, inconvenient, costly, difficult to control and/or when the risk of injury seems rather remote. However, the application of passive strategies is not always possible and even the safest vehicles, agents, etc., can be dangerous in the hands of individuals who behave without regard for their own safety or that of other people. Legal requirements can help in such situations, but again, their application is limited. Thus, there is no substitute for mass education, in addition to the passive strategies outlined above, in the area of injury control.

Summary and conclusions

The second half of this century has witnessed an unprecedented change in health attitudes. It is hard to imagine that until the early

1960s, people believed that they could smoke, eat and drink excessively with nothing worse to fear than a smoker's cough, being a bit overweight or having a hangover. This era of happy ignorance ended in 1964 with the first Surgeon General's report on the dangers of cigarette smoking and the condemnation of food high in cholesterol.

For some time sex appeared be the one behavior that could be enjoyed with impunity, especially after the invention of the pill. This happy state of affairs was first marred by the genital herpes scare (a sexually transmitted viral infection which received wide publicity in the mid-1980s) and ended with the news of the sexual transmission of the AIDS virus. Exercise had always been considered healthy (like eating an apple a day), but only recently has this belief been supported by scientific evidence.

As the proponents of health promotion like to emphasize, the dissemination of the evidence from epidemiological research on the health impact of various health behaviors to the public resulted in substantial attitude and behavior change. Gluttony went out of fashion. Perrier-drinking, vegetarian, monogamous, non-smokers who jog regularly and never drive without wearing their seatbelts have become almost the modal men and women of the post-modern age.

As we have seen, however, there are two ways to evaluate the evidence of the impact of health promotion on health behavior. We can be elated about the 20 per cent reduction in the number of smokers in the USA in the 20 years after the first report on smoking by the Surgeon General in 1964, but we can also be disenchanted by the fact that one-third of the adult population in the USA still smokes cigarettes, despite all the research findings establishing smoking as a health hazard.

How can we explain this apparent lack of response to health warnings? Are they suicidal? Does their resistance to persuasion suggest that health promotion is ineffective and should be abandoned? We would argue that the dramatic changes in health attitudes and behaviors that have occurred over the last 40 years should be sufficient evidence that health education can be effective. One has to keep in mind that, even though good health and a long life are important goals for most persons, they are not the only goals. As Becker (1976) succinctly stated, a person may be a heavy smoker or so committed to work as to omit all exercise, not out of ignorance, but because the life-span forfeited does not seem worth the cost of giving up smoking or working less intensely. Furthermore, whereas public health scientists look at the number of lives that could be saved in the total population if a given behavioral risk factor was eliminated, individuals focus on the *personal* risk they run when engaging in certain health behaviors. Thus, the traffic safety promotion of seatbelts may have been successful in convincing people that thousands of lives could be saved in car crashes if everybody wore seatbelts, but it may have failed to persuade the majority of drivers and passengers that the risk of having an accident at any given time was high enough to justify the effort.

In conclusion, if we want to induce people to change certain health-impairing behaviors, we have to convince them that engaging in these behaviors is associated with a high degree of personal risk which would be considerably reduced if they changed. If we want to change behavior patterns which are not associated with high personal risk but are widely prevalent in a population, we have to implement changes in the incentive structure in addition to employing educational campaigns. Finally, the use of clinical intervention only comes into question when people really want to change their behavior but feel unable to do so on their own.

Suggestions for further reading

Christophersen, E.R. (1989). Injury control. *American Psychologist*, **44,** 237–41. Reviews the research evidence on the effectiveness of the major approaches to injury control.

Fisher, J.D. and Fisher, W.A. (1992). Changing Aids-risk behavior. *Psychological Bulletin*, **111,** 455–74. A comprehensive and critical review of research on interventions aimed at reducing sexual risk behavior.

Kaplan, R.M. (1988). The value dimension in studies of health promotion. In S. Spacapan and S. Oskamp (Eds), *The social psychology of health*. Beverly Hills, CA: Sage. In this readable chapter Kaplan argues that healthy eating is unlikely to prolong our lives.

Paffenbarger, R.S., Jr, Wing, A.L. and Hyde, R.T. (1978). Physical activity as an index of heart attack risk in college alumni. *American Journal of Epidemiology*, **108,** 161–75. Reports one of the classic studies on the relationship between exercise and health.

$\Big/6\Big/$ STRESS AND HEALTH

This chapter and Chapter 7 focus on stress as a risk factor for ill health and on social and personality variables as moderators of the stress–health relationship. There is ample evidence that stress results in health impairment. Although these health consequences are to some extent mediated by changes in the endocrine, immune and autonomic nervous systems, the experience of stress also causes negative changes in health behavior that contribute to the stress–illness relationship. Furthermore, stress is often the result of people's lifestyles. Thus, behavioral factors contribute in a major way to the impact of stress on health. The present chapter examines the evidence for the assumption that stress increases the risk of ill health and discusses some of the processes that might mediate the stress–illness relationship. Chapter 7 then looks at social and personality variables that moderate the impact of stress on health.

Physiological stress and the breakdown of adaptation

The stress concept has been made popular by Selye's seminal work on a pattern of bodily responses that occurs when an organism is exposed to a stressor such as intensive heat or infection. Although much of the theoretical foundation for this work had been prepared by Cannon (1929), Selye's research advanced our understanding of physiological reactions to noxious stimuli and served as a paradigm for later conceptions of stress.

In his highly readable book, *The Stress of Life*, Selye (1976) described how, as a young medical student at the University of

Prague, he was impressed by the fact that, apart from the small number of symptoms characteristic of a given illness (and important for the clinical diagnosis of that illness), there appeared to be many signs of bodily distress which were common to most, if not all, diseases (e.g. loss of weight and appetite, diminished muscular strength, motivational deficits). But it was not until 10 years later, while doing physiological work on animals, that Selye discovered a set of apparently non-specific bodily responses which seemed to occur whenever an organism was exposed to a stressor, whether this stressor was surgical injury, extreme cold, or non-lethal injections of toxic fluids. These bodily reactions consisted of a considerable enlargement of the adrenal cortex, a shrinkage of the thymus and lymph glands, and ulceration of the stomach and duodenum.

The adrenals are two small endocrine glands situated above the kidneys. They consist of two portions – a central part, the medulla, and an outer rind, the cortex. Both synthesize hormones that are involved in mobilizing the organism for action. The thymicolymphatic system, on the other hand, plays an important role in the immune defense of the body. Using these morphological changes as indices of adrenal cortical activity, including an involvement of the immune system, Selye suggested that these endocrine responses helped the organism to cope physiologically with the stressor agent. If we assume that bodily injuries frequently occur in a context in which the animal has to fight or run, physiological responses that mobilize the organism for action are indeed adaptive. Selye defined these non-specific responses as "stress".

No organism can remain in a heightened state of arousal indefinitely. Reactions to stressors therefore change over time. Selye argued that with repeated exposure to the stressor, the defense reaction of the organism passes through three identifiable stages. Together these stages represent the General Adaptation Syndrome. First, in the "alarm" phase, the organism becomes mobilized to meet the threat. In the second stage, "resistance", the organism seems to have adapted to the stressor and the general activation subsides. However, an extended exposure to the same stressor can "exhaust" the adaptive energy of the body. Thus, the third stage, "exhaustion", occurs if the organism fails to overcome the threat and depletes its physiological resources in the process.

There are therefore two ways in which the stressor can harm an organism: It can either cause damage directly if it exceeds the power of adaptation of an organism, or indirectly as a result of the processes marshaled in defense against the stressor. Selye termed the diseases in whose development the stress responses of the organism played a major role, "diseases of adaptation". For example, the ulcers which are typical of the third stage of the general adaptation syndrome would be considered a disease of adaptation. Similarly, the various illnesses which seem to be related to the accumulation of stressful life-events would also belong in this category. Thus, illness is the price the organism has to pay for the defense against extended exposure to stressor agents.

Over the years, Selye's model has been criticized for a number of reasons. One major point of criticism has been that it assigns a very limited role to psychological factors. In contrast to Selye, researchers now believe that psychological appraisal is important in the determination of stress (Lazarus and Folkman 1984). It is possible that even with the stressors used by Selye, the stress response is mediated by emotional disturbance, discomfort and pain rather than being a direct physiological response to the tissue damage caused by these noxious stimuli. Thus, Mason (1975: 24) noted that "conventional laboratory situations designed for the study of physical stressors, such as exercise, heat, cold, etc. very often also elicit an appreciable degree of emotional disturbance, discomfort, and even pain". If precautions are taken to minimize psychological reactions, there is no activation of the adrenal system. A related criticism concerned Selye's "non-specificity assumption" that all stressors produce the same bodily response. There is increasing evidence that specific stressors produce distinct endocrinological responses and that individuals' responses to stress may be influenced by their personalities, perception and biological constitution (Mason 1975; Lazarus and Folkman 1984). These findings challenge Selye's assumption of the uniform response to stress. But this critique should not detract from the fact that Selye's ideas have had a lasting impact on stress research.

Psychosocial stress and health

The second major impetus in the advancement of stress theory came from psychiatrists, who began to study life-events as factors contributing to the development of a variety of psychosomatic and psychiatric illnesses (e.g. Cobb and Lindemann 1943; Holmes and Masuda 1974). Basic to this work is the assumption that psychosocial stress leads to the same bodily changes which Selye observed as a result of tissue damage. This essentially psychosomatic tradition generated clinical and epidemiological research, which tends to support the assumption that the experience of stressful life-events increases the risk of morbidity and even mortality.

The assumption that psychosocial stress had a negative impact on health was first studied in the context of major life-events. Major life-events range from cataclysmic events such as the death of a spouse or being fired from a job to more mundane but still problematic events such as having trouble with one's boss. While some research has examined the impact of *specific* life-events such as bereavement (for a review, see Stroebe and Stroebe 1987) or unemployment (for a review, see Fryer 1988), the majority of studies have used self-report lists of critical life-events to investigate the *cumulative* health-impact of the number or total severity of stressful life-events which subjects reported having experienced during a given period of time (e.g. Holmes and Masuda 1974). More recently, attention has also been focused on the cumulative effect of more minor stressful events or daily hassles on health and illness (e.g. Kanner *et al.* 1981; Monroe 1983). Such hassles might include having too many meetings or not enough time for one's family. The following section will evaluate the evidence from this research with regard to the health-impairing nature of psychosocial stress.

The health impact of cumulative life stress

Major life-events
Self-report scales of critical life-events were pioneered by Holmes and Rahe (1967) with the development of the Schedule of Recent Experiences (SRE) and the Social Readjustment Rating Scale (SRRS). Although there are now a number of second-generation scales – for example, the Life Events Inventory (LES: Sarason *et al.* 1978) and the Psychiatric Epidemiology Research Interview (PERI: Dohrenwend *et al.* 1978), most of the early research on the impact of cumulative life stress on health used the measures of Holmes and Rahe (1967).

Self-report measures typically consist of lists of life-events and require subjects to indicate which of these events they have experienced during a given time period. The checklist developed by

Holmes and Rahe (1967) lists 43 items which describe "life change events". Life change events were defined as those events that require a certain amount of social readjustment from the individual (Table 6.1). Since it was assumed that any event which forced an individual to deviate from his or her habitual pattern would be stressful, the list included pleasant as well as unpleasant events. The inclusion of positive as well as negative changes is reasonable, if, true to the Selye tradition, stress is assumed to be caused by the need to adapt to new situations. However, there is now evidence (e.g. Vinokur and Selzer 1975; Ross and Mirowsky 1979) that only negative events are related to indicators of ill health.

In answering the checklist, subjects are requested to indicate all the life-events they have experienced during a given time period. The measure of cumulative life stress can either consist of the number of life-events experienced during a given period of time (SRE) or of a weighted score that also takes account of the severity of these events (SSRS). Thus the two scales differ only in the weight assigned to life-events. The SSRS provides scale values based on a rating of the magnitude of social readjustment such an event would require (Holmes and Rahe 1967). The unweighted scores (reflecting merely the number of stressful events experienced) or the life change unit scores (reflecting the summed intensity of these events) can then be related to subsequent periods of illness. Surprisingly, weighting scores by the severity of life-events rather than using the mere frequency of events does not seem to improve the power of these scales to predict health problems (L. Cohen 1988).

Although the checklist was also used in a great number of studies in which life-events were only assessed retrospectively after the onset of some illness (e.g. Rahe and Lind 1971; Rahe and Paasikivi 1971), the ease with which it could be administered made it feasible to screen large numbers of people and thus encouraged investigators to conduct prospective studies (i.e. studies in which life-events were assessed before the onset of illness). In one of the most impressive projects of this kind, Rahe (1968) assessed the changes that occurred in the lives of 2500 Navy officers and enlisted men in the 6 months prior to tours of duty aboard three navy cruisers. These life change unit scores were then related to shipboard medical records at the end of the 6 month tour of duty. Individuals with life change unit scores in the top 30 per cent of the distribution were categorized as a high-risk group, those with the lowest 30 per cent as a low-risk group. Rahe found that in the

Table 6.1 The Social Readjustment Rating Scale

Rank	Life-event	Mean value
1	Death of spouse	100
2	Divorce	73
3	Marital separation	65
4	Jail term	63
5	Death of close family member	63
6	Personal injury or illness	53
7	Marriage	50
8	Fired at work	47
9	Marital reconciliation	45
10	Retirement	45
11	Change in health of family member	44
12	Pregnancy	40
13	Sex difficulties	39
14	Gain of new family member	39
15	Business readjustment	39
16	Change in financial state	38
17	Death of close friend	37
18	Change to different line of work	36
19	Change in number of arguments with spouse	35
20	Mortgage over US$10,000	31
21	Foreclosure of mortgage or loan	30
22	Change in responsibilities at work	29
23	Son or daughter leaving home	29
24	Trouble with in-laws	29
25	Outstanding personal achievement	28
26	Wife begin or stop work	26
27	Begin or end school	26
28	Change in living conditions	25
29	Revision of personal habits	24
30	Trouble with boss	23
31	Change in work hours or conditions	20
32	Change in residence	20
33	Change in schools	20
34	Change in recreation	19
35	Change in church activities	19
36	Change in social activities	18
37	Mortgage or loan less than US$10,000	17
38	Change in sleeping habits	16
39	Change in number of family get-togethers	15
40	Change in eating habits	15
41	Vacation	13
42	Christmas	12
43	Minor violations of the law	11

Source: Holmes and Rahe (1967).

first few months of the cruise, the high-risk group had nearly 90 per cent more first illnesses than the low-risk group. Furthermore, the high-risk group consistently reported more illnesses each month for the period of the cruise than did the low-risk group.

However, other prospective studies were less supportive of the stress–illness relationship. Thus, Theorell *et al.* (1975), who studied a sample of over 4000 Swedish construction workers, found no relationship between stressful life-events for a given year and mortality, hospitalization or days off work the following year. Goldberg and Comstock (1976) were similarly unsuccessful in a prospective study relating life-events to death and hospitalization in two American communities. Furthermore, as Rabkin and Struening (1976) pointed out, the correlations between life stress and illness are typically below 0.30, suggesting that life-events account for less than 9 per cent of the variance in illness.

Thus, the initial excitement with which the development of these measures had been greeted was soon followed by a period of critical re-evaluation. One line of argument has raised the possibility that the relationship between life stress and health could be due to a reporting bias (e.g. Mechanic 1978). After all, studies that rely on life-event scales do not assess the amount of stress and the number of illnesses directly, but relate self-reported life stress to treatment-seeking behavior. Thus, individuals with low treatment-seeking thresholds, who consult their doctors for even the most minor health problems, may also be more likely to report any upheaval as a major life-event. This assumption could account for most of the results of the Navy study of Rahe (1968). Although there is evidence that cumulative life stress is positively related to a self-report measure of depression even if reporting bias is controlled by using only those life-events that had been confirmed by a close friend of the subject (Lakey and Heller 1985), such findings do not completely rule out the possibility of reporting bias. It is plausible that individuals who are more depressed may also be more likely to talk to their friends about their negative experience.

Along similar lines, Watson and Pennebaker (1989) argued that self-report measures of both stressful life-events and health complaints reflect a pervasive mood disposition of negative affectivity, which represents a stable personality disposition to experience negative mood and is closely related to the dimension of neuroticism. While negative affectivity correlates highly with measures of symptom reporting, it seems to be unrelated to objective health indicators (e.g. blood pressure levels, serum risk factors, immune system functions). Watson and Pennebaker (1989) suggest that individuals who score high on negative affectivity are hypervigilant and are therefore more likely to notice and attend to normal body sensations. Since their scanning is fraught with anxiety and uncertainty, they tend to interpret normal symptoms as painful and pathological.

Another critical argument against the use of self-report measures of life-events has been that of the contamination of stress and illness measures (e.g. Schroeder and Costa 1984). Life-event scales may be confounded with measures of health in at least two ways. First, life-event scales frequently include items that may reflect the physical and psychological conditions of the respondent. If items such as "personal injury or illness" or "pregnancy" are used as measures of stressful life-events, then the event score is directly contaminated with concurrent physical health. Second, life-event scales often include items that could reflect the result rather than the cause of psychological problems (e.g. troubles with in-laws, being fired at work, separation). Consistent with these assumptions, Schroeder and Costa (1984) demonstrated that the correlation obtained between standard measures of life-events and physical illness disappeared when "contaminated items" were eliminated from the life-event scale. However, these findings could not be replicated by Maddi et al. (1987).

Minor life-events

These methodological problems increase in severity as we move from self-report measures of major life-events to scales that assess minor events such as "daily hassles". Hassles are "irritating, frustrating, distressing demands that to some degree characterize everyday transactions with the environment" (Kanner et al. 1981: 3). Examples of events that can be hassles are misplacing and losing things, concerns about new events, traffic, being lonely or not getting enough sleep. Kanner et al. (1981) developed a Hassles Scale that consists of a list of 117 potential hassles. Subjects are asked to mark each hassle that has happened to them during a given period of time and then to indicate how severe each of the hassles had been during this time (somewhat severe, moderately severe, extremely severe). From this information, two summary scores can be computed: (1) *frequency*, reflecting the number of items checked, and (2) *intensity*, reflecting the mean severity of the items checked. Examples of hassles are listed in Table 6.2.

Table 6.2 Example items from the Hassles Scale

1 Misplacing or losing things	16 Smoking too much
2 Troublesome neighbors	17 Use of alcohol
3 Social obligations	18 Personal use of drugs
4 Inconsiderate smokers	19 Too many responsibilities
5 Troubling thoughts about your future	20 Decisions about having children
6 Thoughts about death	21 Non-family members living in your house
7 Health of a family member	
8 Not enough money for clothing	22 Care for pet
9 Not enough money for housing	23 Planning meals
	24 Concerned about the meaning of life
10 Concerns about owing money	25 Trouble relaxing
11 Concerns about getting credit	26 Trouble making decisions
12 Concerns about money for emergencies	27 Problems getting along with fellow workers
13 Someone owes you money	28 Customers or clients give you a hard time
14 Financial responsibility for someone who doesn't live with you	29 Home maintenance (inside)
	30 Concerns about job security
15 Cutting down on electricity, water, etc.	31 Concerns about retirement
	32 Laid-off or out of work

Source: Kanner *et al.* (1981).

In one study, the Hassles Scale was given to 100 middle-aged adults for 9 consecutive months and related to reported psychological symptoms, including depression and anxiety (Kanner *et al.* 1981). Hassles were found to be a better predictor of concurrent and subsequent psychological symptoms than were more major life-events. Furthermore, while major life-events had little impact on symptoms independent of the effect of hassles, hassles continued to predict symptoms, even after the impact of major life-events had been statistically controlled. That hassles predicted health outcome as well or better than major life-events was also reported by DeLongis *et al.* (1982), Monroe (1983), Weinberger *et al.* (1987) and Zarski (1984).

Research using the Hassles Scale was soon subjected to the same criticism that had been levelled against studies that relied on measures of major life-events. Specifically, the Dohrenwends and their colleagues raised the issue of contamination (Dohrenwend *et al.* 1984; Dohrenwend and Shrout 1985). They first argued that the Hassles Scale contained many items that may well reflect psychological symptoms (e.g. "You have had sexual problems other than those resulting from physical problems"; "You are concerned about your use of alcohol"; "You have had a fear of rejection"). When Lazarus *et al.* (1985) demonstrated that a hassles subscale consisting only of items that were apparently unconfounded showed as high a correlation with psychological symptoms as a subscale that consisted mainly of confounded items, Dohrenwend and Shrout (1985) changed their argument to suggest that all hassles reflected symptoms, due to the response format of the Hassles Scale. They argued that the fact that the lowest intensity permitted by the response scale is "somewhat severe" could be interpreted by subjects as implying that an event had to be at least "somewhat severe" to be reported as a hassle. Thus, only subjects who experienced difficulties in coping with a given hassle would feel that they should report it.

In a defense of the Hassles Scale, Reich *et al.* (1988) criticized this reasoning. While they agreed that the intensity score was likely to reflect the more subjective response tendency of the individual (i.e. symptoms), they argued that the frequency score should be interpreted as reflecting the more "objective source of stress". Reich *et al.* (1988) showed that the two scores had a very low correlation with each other and were both independently related to health problems. However, as in the case of major life-events, the assumption that number of hassles is an indicator of objective sources of stress is called into question by findings reported by Watson and Pennebaker (1989) that both hassles scores were significantly correlated with a measure of negative affectivity. Furthermore, when variation in negative affectivity was statistically controlled in a hierarchical multiple regression, hassles had a much reduced impact on health complaints and accounted for only 2–6 per cent of the variance.

Conclusions

There is evidence that measures of cumulative stress, reflecting both major and minor stressors, are significantly related to psychological and physical health problems. However, there is now considerable doubt about how justifiable it is to interpret this relationship in terms of a causal impact of stress on health. There are not only the problems of reporting biases and item contamination, but there is also increasing evidence that self-report measures of both stress and health complaints reflect a stable personality disposition of negative affectivity, or neuroticism, that could at least be partly responsible for the relationship observed between these measures. To alleviate these doubts, any further research that employs self-report measures of cumulative stress should at least try to use objective indicators of health status.

The health impact of specific life-events: The case of marital bereavement

Most of the ambiguities involved in using self-report measures of stress can be avoided by studying the health consequences of specific stressful life-events. Marital bereavement combines a number of features which make it particularly suited to the study of the health impact of stressful life-events. Marital bereavement is not only one of the most severely stressful life-events, it is also objectifiable (thereby eliminating the risk of reporting biases affecting the measure of stress). Since marital bereavement is also reflected in census and health records, large bodies of data are available which permit the analysis of excess risk in terms of specific illnesses and even mortality. Finally, with the exception of loss due to suicide of the partner, there can be no doubt about the temporal priority of the stressful life-event. Thus, while many of the life-events such as divorce or separation typically listed in life-event inventories could be consequences rather than the cause of personality problems or depression, this is unlikely in the case of bereavement. We will therefore present a brief overview of the major findings of research on the health consequences of marital bereavement.

The loss of a spouse through death can indeed adversely affect the health of the surviving partner. This has been shown both in epidemiological surveys comparing marital status groups on various health measures, and in longitudinal cohort studies examining the health status of bereaved (compared with non-bereaved) persons for a period of time following loss (for reviews, see Osterweis *et al.* 1984; Parkes 1986; Stroebe and Stroebe 1987; Stroebe *et al.* 1993).

Consequences can be so direct that the life of the bereaved

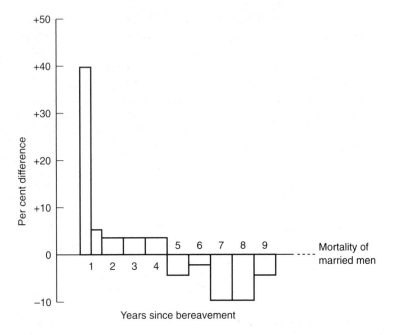

Figure 6.1 Percentage difference between the mortality rates of
widowers over age 54 and those of married men of the same age by
number of years since bereavement
Source: Parkes *et al.* (1969)

person is itself threatened. As cross-sectional surveys in many different countries have shown, the widowed have higher mortality
rates than their married counterparts. Furthermore, the greatest
risk to life appears to be in the first few weeks and months following loss. The classic study by Parkes *et al.* (1969) clearly illustrates this phenomenon. As Figure 6.1. shows, in their longitudinal
study of a sample of widowers over the age of 54, there was a
40 per cent increase in mortality during the first 6 months of
bereavement, compared with married controls over an equivalent
period. Although there are some variations between studies in
patterns of excess rates for the widowed, certain regularities have
emerged (for a review, see M. Stroebe and W. Stroebe 1993).
Thus, excesses for widowers are relatively higher than those for
widows, as are the excesses for younger compared with older
bereaved spouses.

Despite the excess risk of mortality, expressed in absolute numbers, there are very few bereaved persons who do actually die prematurely. However, for a much larger proportion, bereavement is associated not only with intense suffering over an extended period of time, but also with an increased risk of succumbing to a variety of psychological and somatic complaints and illnesses. Thus, depression rates are higher for widowed than non-widowed persons. Visits to physicians are more frequent among the former than the latter, and the physical illness rates of the bereaved are elevated.

Studies are beginning to identify those bereaved individuals who are at particular risk of suffering from the various adverse consequences of loss. There is some evidence (for a review, see Sanders 1993) that health consequences are affected by such factors as the mode of death (more severe consequences after a sudden rather than an expected loss), gender (men suffering more severe consequences) and the extent of social support the individual receives after the loss (more severe consequences for people who do not receive much social support).

While the relationship between bereavement and various mental and physical health debilities has been reasonably well established, this alone is not convincing evidence that it is the stress of bereavement that is the mediating factor. There are a number of alternative explanations. Depression models would tend to look instead to such factors as loneliness consequent upon losing a loved person, to reactions of helplessness and "giving up". Others have argued in terms of artifacts, such as homogamy between spouses (i.e. the similarity of marital partners in sociological, psychological and physical traits), or the fact that partners had joint unfavorable environments (e.g. they breathed the same unhealthy air or both had poor diets).

However, there also seems very little doubt that bereavement is stressful. Longitudinal studies have consistently identified a variety of strains associated with the loss of a spouse, ranging from financial hardships to social constraints to problems in the care of bereaved children (Stroebe *et al.* 1993). The results that were outlined above in relation to risk factors for poor bereavement outcome (low self-esteem, lack of social support, a sudden loss, etc.) can easily be interpreted within a stress framework. Thus, traumatic deaths are particularly difficult for survivors to come to terms with, and are associated with high rates of debility (Raphael 1986). That such circumstances are more stressful for survivors than the peaceful death of an elderly person "in the fullness of time" seems self-evident. Moreover, such results suggest that it is persons with inadequate coping resources – for example, those people who hold the belief that they have little control over events – who feel particularly unable to cope with the stressful circumstances of bereavement (W. Stroebe and M. Stroebe 1993).

What makes critical life-events stressful?

By relating the incidence of illness to specific stressful events, research on the health impact of critical life-events evaded the thorny issue of specifying why certain psychological experiences are stressful, how the organism recognizes stressful events and distinguishes them from positive events, and how inter-individual differences in reactions to stress can be explained. Thus, while it appears quite plausible that the physical stressors used by Selye, such as extreme cold or the injection of non-lethal amounts of toxic fluids, should challenge the defense systems of an organism, it is less obvious why the death of a partner or the loss of a job should have a similar impact.

These issues have been addressed by psychological approaches to stress which analyze the cognitive processes that mediate between life-events and stress. Interactional approaches take the general view that stress is the result of a perceived mismatch between environmental demands and the resources available to the individual in dealing with these demands (e.g. French and Kahn 1962; Lazarus and Folkman 1984). A more specific theory developed by Seligman and his colleagues (Seligman 1975; Abramson et al. 1978; Peterson and Seligman 1987) identified perceived lack of control as a key characteristic of stressful situations.

Stress as a person–environment interaction

For several decades, Lazarus (e.g. Lazarus and Folkman 1984) has been the chief proponent of the interactional view of stress. According to his widely accepted definition, "Psychological stress is a particular relationship between the person and the environment that is appraised by the individual as taxing or exceeding his or her resources and endangering his or her well-being" (Lazarus and Folkman 1984: 19). Thus, the extent of the stress experienced in a given situation neither depends solely on the demands of the situation nor on the resources of the person but on the relationship between demands and resources as perceived (appraised) by the individual. This is not meant to imply, however, that situations do not differ in the extent to which they are likely to be experienced as stressful.

The two central processes in Lazarus' theory that determine the extent of stress experiences in a given situation are cognitive appraisal and coping. *Cognitive appraisal* is an evaluative process which determines why and to what extent a particular situation is perceived as stressful by a given individual. Lazarus distinguishes three basic forms of appraisal: primary appraisal, secondary appraisal and reappraisal. In *primary appraisal*, individuals categorize a given situation with respect to its significance for their well-being and decide whether the situation is irrelevant, positive or stressful.

A situation is appraised as stressful if it implies harm/loss, threat, or challenge. Once a situation has been categorized as stressful, individuals have to evaluate their coping options to decide which strategy will be most effective in a given situation in achieving the intended outcome. Thus, a driver who runs into ice and fog on a highway has to decide whether to go on as before, to drive more slowly, or even to stop at the next parking place to wait for conditions to improve. This assessment of coping resources and options is referred to as *secondary appraisal*. The extent of stress experienced in a given situation depends on the combination of primary appraisal of what is at stake and secondary appraisal of coping options.

The notion of *reappraisal* was introduced to emphasize that cognitive appraisal processes are in a permanent state of flux, due to new inputs. Thus, the original appraisal of a situation may change as new information about the situation or about the impact of one's own behavior is received. The realization that one is quite able to cope with the difficult driving conditions or that what one thought was ice was in fact only wetness will lead to a reappraisal of the threat caused by poor driving conditions.

When a situation has been appraised as stressful, individuals have to do something to master the situation and/or to control their emotional reactions to the situation. These processes of responding to stressful demands have been called *coping processes*. Lazarus and Folkman (1984) distinguish two basic forms of coping, problem-focused coping and emotion-focused coping. Coping is *problem-focused* when it is directed at managing and altering the problem that is causing distress. For example, a student who is worried about an impending exam will do everything to be well-prepared (e.g. attend classes, join a work group). However, the student might also be so anxious that he or she begins to have trouble sleeping or is unable to concentrate. In order to reduce this emotional distress, the student may engage in a range of *emotion-focused* forms of coping. These could include cognitive operations such as attempts to reappraise the situation as less threatening. But they may also include actions such as taking sleeping pills, smoking or drinking alcohol in order to cope with the emotional distress and calm one's nerves.

The extent to which the situation is experienced as stressful, as well as the individual's success in mastering it, will depend on his or her *coping resources*. Lazarus and Folkman (1984) distinguish resources that are primarily properties of the person and resources that are primarily environmental. The person-resources include physical resources such as health and energy, psychological resources such as positive beliefs (e.g. positive self-concept, belief in control) and competencies such as problem-solving and social skills. Examples of environmental resources are material resources (e.g. money) and social support.

The cognitive stress model developed by Lazarus and his colleagues offers a general framework for the analysis of psychological stress. However, although the model identifies many important general principles of stress and coping, its high level of generality can be a disadvantage in research that attempts to use the model to derive testable predictions for specific stressful life-events. Therefore, a number of more specific stress theories have been developed that either apply the interactive approach to specific life-events (e.g. the Deficit Model of Bereavement: Stroebe and Stroebe 1987; the Person–Environment Fit Model of work stress: Caplan 1983) and/or specify more accurately those aspects of a situation that determine the intensity and persistence of the stress experience (e.g. the Theory of Learned Helplessness: Seligman 1975). We will focus on the theory of learned helplessness because it has equalled the model of Lazarus as a major influence on stress research.

Stress as learned helplessness

Although Seligman's (1975) interest was in the causes of depression rather than stress ("stress" does not appear as a term in the subject index of his 1975 book), his analysis of the conditions under which life-events can result in depression identified perceived lack of control as an essential characteristic of situations that are stressful. The original formulation of the learned helplessness model was derived from escape–avoidance research conducted with animals. These experiments showed that while normal animals, exposed to electric shocks which they can escape, learn to escape after a few shocks, animals that had previously experienced unavoidable shock do not seem to learn the escape response. Later research demonstrated that repeated experiences of uncontrollability had similar effects on humans (e.g. Hiroto 1974; Hiroto and Seligman 1975).

Seligman developed the learned helplessness model as a unified theoretical framework which integrated the data from animal as well as human research. The basic assumption is that when people or animals experience an event that they cannot control, they develop an expectation of lack of control in similar situations. This learning results in the helplessness syndrome, which consists of motivational, cognitive and emotional deficits. If the persons or animals have learned that the escape from aversive stimulation occurs independent of responses, they will not try very hard to initiate a response that can produce relief; they will also fail to learn new responses that would help them to avoid aversive outcomes and they will react to the traumatic experience first with fear and then depression. On the basis of the similarity of the symptoms of learned helplessness and depression, Seligman proposed that learned helplessness was a major cause of reactive depression.

The extension of the learned helplessness model to depression raised a number of problems. Seligman (1975) had originally emphasized that it was the uncontrollability rather than the aversiveness of outcomes which was responsible for the motivational and emotional deficits. It seemed implausible, however, that people would get depressed because uncontrollable good things tended to happen to them. Furthermore, the view that depressive persons feel helpless is inconsistent with their tendency toward self-blame. If individuals believe that their outcomes are independent

of their responses, how could depressed individuals feel responsible for these outcomes? Another inadequacy of the old helplessness model concerned the generality of helplessness across situations
and duration over time (Abramson *et al.* 1978). The model does
not permit predictions about the conditions under which uncontrollability leads to long-term and broadly generalized helplessness
symptoms, compared with such experiences that result in temporary helplessness that may only concern a very restricted sphere of
life (Försterling 1988).

To solve these problems, a cognitive revision of the model was
suggested by Abramson *et al.* (1978). According to the revised
model, the relation between the experience of uncontrollability
and depressive symptoms is mediated by individuals' causal attributions, that is, their interpretations of the reasons for their failure
to control a given situation, which implies aversive outcomes
(Abramson *et al.* 1978). There are three attributional dimensions
assumed to be important in producing helplessness: internality,
stability and globality. For example, a person who loses his or her
job might have reasons to attribute this either internally (e.g.
personal incompetence) or externally (bankruptcy of the firm he
or she worked for). While he or she might feel depressed in either
situation, the attribution to personal incompetence is most likely
to result in loss of self-esteem. Personal incompetence would also
be a more stable cause than a bankruptcy. While it is unlikely that
a future employer would also have to close down, personal incompetence is a stable condition that would also be a problem with
the next employer. Globality refers to the extent to which helplessness is confined to specific areas. For example, if an individual
merely felt incompetent with regard to a very specific line of work,
and that he or she would do much better by changing to another
line, helplessness would be much less pervasive than if the individual felt generally incompetent to work in his or her chosen
occupation. Finally, the severity and intensity of depressive symptoms will be the greater, the more important and potentially aversive
the situation is in which helplessness is experienced.

Thus, according to the attributional theory of learned helplessness, it is not the aversiveness of a negative life-event that results
in stress and depression, but rather the experience of lack of control induced by negative events that are attributed to internal,
stable and global causes. The pre-helplessness phase, in which the
individual expends effort to bring the situation under control, is

characterized by ongoing stress. During this phase, individuals will try to cope with the threat, either by problem-focused coping or by emotion-focused coping. Learned helplessness, when the individual stops trying to cope, is analogous to the phase of exhaustion of resources described by Selye. People often do recover and manage to re-establish control. But the more the individual attributes the helplessness to internal, stable and global causes, the more the stressful experience will result in enduring depressive reactions with the associated cognitive and emotional consequences.

The attributional model further suggested that a characteristic *attributional style* may exist that disposes individuals toward reacting with depression to stressful life-events. Seligman and colleagues (e.g. Abramson *et al.* 1978) argued that depression-prone individuals would tend to attribute aversive events to internal, global and stable causes. Two measures of this pessimistic explanatory style were developed: a self-report questionnaire called the Attributional Style Questionnaire (ASQ) and a content analysis procedure called the CAVE (Content Analysis of Verbatim Explanations) technique.

The ASQ presents respondents with six bad events (e.g. you meet a friend who acts hostilely toward you) and six good events (e.g. you did a project which is highly praised). Respondents are asked to imagine themselves in these situations and to provide causal explanations for these events. They are then required to rate each cause in terms of internality, stability and globality. Explanatory style is inferred from the respondents' scores across the three attributional dimensions, computing separate averages for good and bad events. With the CAVE technique, verbatim quotes of causal attributions for good or bad events of the sample of interest are rated by judges in terms of their internality, stability and globality. This technique allows researchers to assess attributional style on the basis of interview material collected for a completely different purpose.

The relationship between attributional style and depression has been observed in numerous studies. Thus, a meta-analysis of more than 100 studies found moderate correlations between the predicted attributional pattern and depression (Sweeney *et al.* 1986). However, critics of the revised theory of learned helplessness doubt the importance of attributions as mediators of depression. In particular, Brewin (1988) argued that some events may have such a major impact on their own account that causal cognitions are relatively unimportant in mediating the emotional response. Thus, there are life-events which are so far beyond the range of usual human experience that they would be markedly distressing to almost anyone; for example, extreme situations such as the result of acts of war, collective disasters and accidents, crimes of violence, the violent loss of a loved one. And yet while powerful events such as the loss of a child or spouse are stressful and saddening for nearly everybody, only a minority of those affected by loss react with enduring depression and health deterioration. It seems plausible that the depressive pattern of attributions is associated with a weakened resistance to and poorer recovery from depression.

In their more recent research, Seligman and colleagues (e.g. Peterson and Seligman 1987; Peterson et al. 1988) have used the CAVE technique to relate the pessimistic attributional style to physical illness and even mortality. In doing so, Seligman addressed an important claim made in his 1975 book, namely that learned helplessness would result in an impairment of physical as well as mental health.

In one study, the age at death of members of the Baseball Hall of Fame whose playing career occurred between 1900 and 1950 was related to their characteristic attributional style (Peterson and Seligman 1987). Attributional style could be assessed for 24 players on the basis of verbatim quotes reported in sports pages. Peterson and Seligman found a marginally significant correlation ($r = 0.26$) between the extent to which players offered internal, stable and global explanations for bad events and life-expectancy. Players who offered external, unstable and specific explanations for good events also lived shorter lives ($r = 0.45$).

In another study, attributional style was assessed from interviews completed at the age of 25 years by 99 graduates of Harvard University from the classes of 1942–44, who were mentally and physically fit at the time of the interview. Men who at age 25 explained bad events by referring to their own internal, stable and global negative qualities had significantly poorer health some 20–35 years later. Thus, health status assessed by the individual's personal physician at age 45 showed a significant correlation of 0.37 with pessimistic explanatory style measured at age 25. Health status measured at age 60 correlated 0.25 with the same attributional style scores. These findings suggest that pessimistic attributional style in early adulthood is a risk factor for poor physical health in middle and late adulthood. However, although Peterson and Seligman (1987) discuss various pathways between explanatory style and physical well-being, there is little empirical evidence about the processes which might mediate this relationship.

Conclusions

Both Lazarus and Seligman developed theories that identify the cognitive processes underlying the stress experience and make predictions with regard to the initiation of coping behaviors. According to the cognitive stress theory of Lazarus, a situation is stressful if it is potentially harmful and if the individual perceives that his or her resources are insufficient to prevent the aversive outcome. While the original theory of learned helplessness conceived of stress as resulting from uncontrollability regardless of whether the event implied harmful or positive outcomes, the stress definition of the revised model is consistent with that of Lazarus and his colleagues in perceiving stress as resulting from the risk of encountering aversive consequences. The revised version of learned helplessness theory further specifies the conditions under which such aversive situations are likely to result in persistent feelings of hopelessness and depression. The theory suggests that perceived lack of control that is attributed to internal, stable and global causes is likely to result in anxiety and depression. The model further assumes that a characteristic attributional style exists which constitutes a risk factor for depression as well as poor physical health.

With regard to coping, both theories imply that when individuals are exposed to potentially threatening situations, they will initiate coping strategies to contain the threat. These strategies might consist of problem-oriented coping behaviors but they could also involve emotion-oriented coping behaviors. In addition, the learned helplessness model makes the prediction that in chronic stress situations, coping activities will essentially be abandoned, if the causes of uncontrollability are perceived as internal, stable and global.

How does psychosocial stress affect health?

Stressful life-events like the loss of a job or the death of a spouse do not operate on one's bodily system in the same manner as the noxious physical or chemical stimuli studied by Selye. And yet, as we saw earlier, there can be little doubt that the experience of stressful life-events is associated with an increased risk of a wide range of physical and mental disorders. There are two types of mechanisms which mediate the impact of psychosocial stress on health: first, stress can affect health directly through changes in the body's physiology; second, stress can affect health indirectly through changes in individual behavior.

Physiological responses to stress

Evolutionarily, the function of physiological reactions to stress appears to have been to prepare the organism for action. If we assume that bodily injuries frequently occur in a context in which an animal has to fight or run, it makes sense that the stress responses consist mainly of catabolic processes, that is, processes involved with expenditure of energy from reserves stored in the body. Therefore, the sympathetic-adrenal-medullary system and the pituitary-adrenocortical system are the two major neuroendocrine systems that are responsible for many of the physiological changes associated with stress.

Activation of the *sympathetic-adrenal-medullary system* leads to an increase in the secretion of two catecholamines, norepinephrine and epinephrine. The release of catecholamines stimulates cardiovascular activity and raises blood pressure. The heart beats faster, increasing the amount of blood pumped with each beat. By constricting peripheral blood vessels and those leading to the gastrointestinal tract, blood pressure is raised. At the same time, the arteries serving muscles (including the coronary arteries of the heart muscle) are dilated, thus increasing their blood supply. Catecholamines also relax air passages. Breathing becomes faster and deeper, the bronchioles of the lungs dilate, and the secretion of mucus in the air passages decreases. Thus, more oxygen is available for the metabolism. Catecholamines also cause the liberation of glucose (one of the major sources of usable energy) from the liver, thus availing the muscles of large energy resources. One further effect, which is quite advantageous in the case of physical injury, is that catecholamines increase the tendency of the blood to coagulate.

The activation of the *pituitary-adrenocortical system* leads to increases in the secretion and release of corticosteroids from the adrenal cortex. For the physiology of stress reactions, the most interesting corticosteroid is cortisol. Cortisol is important for energy mobilization of the body. It promotes the synthesis of glucose from the liver. Cortisol also mobilizes the fat stores from adipose tissues and increases the level of serum lipids – that is, fat-like substances in the blood such as triclycerids and cholesterol – which also provide energy for skeletal and heart muscles.

A second major effect of the increase in cortisol production is its impact on the immune system. Pharmacological doses of cortisol have been shown to cause an atrophy of the lymphoid structures, and thus act to impair the activity of the body's immune system. Since inflammation of the affected areas (one of the painful side-effects of an active immune system) would tend to interfere with fight or flight responses, one could speculate that the prevention of such interference might initially be more important than the destruction of the intruding agent.

Suppression of pain is also helped by endogenous opiates, which are morphine-like peptides that are released in response to stress (O'Leary 1990). Stress-induced opiate activation has been shown to reduce pain reactivity in humans (Bandura et al. 1987). There is some evidence that these endogenous opiates also have a suppressive effect on the immune system (O'Leary 1990).

The activation of these physiological stress systems prepares the organism for combat or escape. However, the vigorous physical activity which the stress response prepares us for is rarely an appropriate response to cope with the typical stressful life-events encountered today. Instead, in many stress situations, the stress response is likely to hinder rather than help coping and adjustment. Furthermore, while stress response in the wild was typically activated by transitory stressors, today many stressors are long-term rather than immediate, resulting in more extended elevations of arousal levels. This can impair the functioning of various organ systems, including the immune system, leaving the organism open to infections.

Behavioral responses to stress

The experience of stress motivates individuals to engage in a variety of behavioral strategies which aim to reduce the threat or to cope with the emotions aroused by the potentially aversive experience.

Table 6.3 Percentage of men and women interviewed who specified an increase in their use of tranquillizers, sleeping tablets, alcoholic beverages or cigarettes[a]

	Women		Men	
	Married (n = 30)	Widowed (n = 30)	Married (n = 30)	Widowed (n = 30)
Tranquillizers	0.0	24.1	0.0	10.0
Sleeping tablets	3.3	13.3	3.3	6.9
Alcoholic beverages	3.3	6.7	3.3	17.2
Smoking	10.0	17.2	10.0	30.0

[a] Data from the first interviews of the Tübingen Longitudinal Study of Bereavement. Widowed respondents were asked for an increase in use since the death of their partner. Married respondents were asked for increases during the comparable time period.

For example, an executive who is competing for an important promotion will attempt to increase chances of success by working longer hours and by generally increasing the quality of his or her performance. When the workload becomes so extensive that people abandon regular meals and just "grab a quick bite" whenever there is time, when they resort to tranquillizers, cigarettes or alcohol to calm down or go to sleep, coping behavior can become deleterious to one's health.

The assumption that individuals who are under stress are more likely to engage in these kinds of unhealthy behavior patterns has been supported by findings from a survey of a probability sample reported by Cohen and Williamson (1988). In this study, small but statistically significant correlations were observed between perceived stress and shorter periods of sleep, infrequent consumption of breakfast, increased quantity of alcohol consumption, and greater frequency of usage of illicit drugs. Marginal relations were also found between stress and (a) smoking and (b) lack of physical exercise.

Similarly, the widows and widowers who participated in the Tübingen Longitudinal Study of Bereavement reported changes in tranquillizer use, smoking and alcohol consumption (Table 6.3). While widows mainly increased their use of tranquillizers and sleeping pills, widowers reported increases in alcohol consumption and smoking. This pattern is consistent with epidemiological data that show cirrhosis of the liver to be one of the causes of death in which widowers show the greatest excess over married men (M. Stroebe and W. Stroebe 1993). It is also consistent with reports from relapsed addicts that stress often immediately preceded their return to drug use (e.g. Condiotte and Lichtenstein 1981; Shiffman 1982; Baer and Lichtenstein 1988; Bliss *et al.* 1989). Behavioral factors such as alcohol use and carelessness probably play a role in the relatively high accident rates of people under stress.

Thus, there is considerable evidence to suggest that the experience of stress is associated with health practices which constitute health risks. Since it appears very plausible that individuals change their health practices as a consequence of the stress experience, these behavioral responses to stress are likely to contribute to the health deterioration that has been observed in people who endure stressful life-events.

Stress and disease

The cost of stress is expressed in terms of its effect on health and well-being. The disorders which have attracted most attention in this respect are infections, coronary heart disease, alimentary conditions such as dyspepsia and ulcers, and psychopathological problems such as depression. Stress has also been suspected to be important for many other diseases, including diabetes mellitus, asthma and even cancer. However, there is still debate about the causal role of stress in the development of various diseases and the mechanisms that mediate this relationship. We will therefore merely illustrate these stress effects using the role of stress in infections and in coronary heart disease as examples.

Stress and infectious disease

Infections are obviously caused by some infectious agent. But exposure to such agents does not always cause infection. There are numerous factors which affect an individual's susceptibility to disease (e.g. prior exposure to the microorganism and the development of immunity, nutritional status of the host, a wide range of genetic factors). Since Selye's classic work on the effect of stress on the immune system, exposure to stress has to be included among the determinants of individual susceptibility.

The general function of the immune system is to identify and eliminate foreign, "non-self", materials that contact or enter the body. These foreign substances, called *antigens*, include bacteria, viruses, tumor cells, toxins, etc. The processes of identification and elimination are accomplished by several different types of lymphocytes (white blood cells). Measurements of immune function typically calculate the number and/or functional abilities of subgroups of lymphocytes. Since these different subgroups perform specialized functions, it is not possible to use a single measure to determine global immunological competence (O'Leary 1990; Laudenslager *et al.* 1993).

There is now empirical support for the assumption that psychosocial stress is associated with an impairment of the functioning of the immune system. Thus, studies of such diverse groups as bereaved spouses, separated and divorced men and women, psychiatric patients with a major depression, and family caregivers of Alzheimer's disease victims have demonstrated that members of such groups are more distressed and show relatively poorer immune functions than well-matched community counterparts (e.g. Stein *et al.* 1985; Kiecolt-Glaser *et al.* 1987, 1988). Other researchers have observed some suppression of immune function in medical students during examinations, compared with 1 month previously when the subjects were less distressed (e.g. Glaser *et al.* 1985). There is also increasing evidence that changes in immune response occur as a function of prolonged and repeated exposure to stress (e.g. Kiecolt-Glaser *et al.* 1987; McKinnon *et al.* 1989). For example, McKinnon *et al.* (1989) found impairment in immune functions (relative to a matched control group) in people who lived near the nuclear power station at Three Mile Island and who had been exposed to more than 6 years of stressful uncertainty associated with the accident at this station.

It is less clear, however, whether these changes in immune function really result in health deterioration. While we know that gross alterations in immunity can be associated with greater morbidity and mortality (e.g. AIDS), little is known about the actual health consequences of these less extreme changes in immune function (Kiecolt-Glaser and Glaser 1991). Although there is now evidence that stress increases the risk that individuals exposed to an infectious agent will develop clinical disease, most comes from studies that use self-reported symptoms or use of health care services as measures of clinical disease (Cohen and Williamson 1991). Only a few studies have prospectively demonstrated a covariation among psychological stressors and actual health changes in the presence of immunologic alterations (e.g. Kasl *et al.* 1979).

Stress and coronary heart disease

There are two major forms of coronary heart disease, namely angina pectoris and myocardial infarction. The symptoms of angina pectoris are periodic attacks of distinctive chest pain, usually situated behind the sternum and radiating to the chest and left shoulder. Attacks of angina pectoris are typically brought on by physical exercise and emotional exertion. They are quickly relieved by rest or medication aimed at dilating blood vessels and reducing blood pressure. The major cause of angina pectoris is an insufficient supply of oxygen to the heart due to atherosclerosis, a thickening of the innermost walls of coronary arteries. This thickening is caused by the formation of plaque. Plaque consists of fatty deposits of excess amounts of serum lipids, especially cholesterol. Attacks of angina pectoris rarely involve permanent damage to the heart muscle, but are a warning that the blood supply to the heart is in some way impaired.

If plaque grows at a rate exceeding the blood supply available for the nutrition of its cells, it is likely to rupture and form the basis for a thrombosis, which will then completely block an already narrow passage. Such ruptures may also be the result of hemodynamic factors such as high levels of arterial blood pressure (Herd 1978). The formation of blood clots which obstruct the artery and diminish the blood supply to the left ventricle of the heart are the most frequent cause of myocardial infarction, a necrosis (death) of the heart tissue caused by a long-lasting insufficiency of the oxygen supply. Myocardial infarction is one of the major causes of death in most industrialized nations.

There are several mechanisms by which stress can contribute to coronary heart disease. Stress is likely to accelerate the development of atherosclerosis by increasing the secretion of catecholamines and cortisol (both involved in mobilizing fat stores) and thus increasing the level of serum lipids. In an extensive review of research on the impact of stress on the level of serum lipids, Dimsdale and Herd (1982) found that the majority of studies showed significant increases in cholesterol and especially free fatty acid levels in response to emotional arousal induced by a variety of stressors. Catecholamines also increase the tendency of blood to coagulate, which may contribute to the formation of blood clots and consequent blocking of arteries, especially arteries already narrowed due to the formation of atherosclerotic plaque. Finally, stress is associated with a number of poor health practices which raise the risk of coronary heart disease. Thus, individuals under stress are likely to increase their consumption of cigarettes and alcohol, adopt poor eating habits and engage in very little physical exercise (Cohen and Williamson 1988).

Much of the evidence for the relationship between stress and coronary heart disease is based on retrospective studies that used life-event scales and are therefore open to methodological criticism (e.g. Rahe and Lind 1971; Rahe and Paasikivi 1971; Theorell and Rahe 1971; Rahe et al. 1974). For example, Rahe and colleagues (1974) gathered life change data on more than 200 survivors of myocardial infarctions and a similar number of cases of abrupt coronary death in Helsinki. Next of kin, most of whom were spouses, provided the life change data for the victims of sudden deaths. The results indicated a marked elevation in the magnitude of total life changes during the months prior to infarction compared with the same time period 1 year earlier. The major problem with this type of study is that the retrospective assessment of life-events is likely to be influenced by the respondent's knowledge of the occurrence of an illness. Since the belief that stress is bad for coronary health is part of common culture, respondents inclined to search for explanations for their own or their partner's illness, are likely to remember more stressful life-events as having occurred just prior to the event.

However, there are now also numerous studies on the impact of stress on heart disease which used prospective designs on individuals who were already at high risk (e.g. Byrne et al. 1981; Ruberman et al. 1984). For example, Byrne et al. (1981) examined a cohort of 120 men and women who survived heart attacks. At the first interview, which took place 10–14 days following their admission into a coronary care unit, these patients responded to an extensive questionnaire that also contained questions about personal, social and financial worries prior to the heart attack which, in the judgment of the patients, may have contributed to the attack. Of the 102 members of the original sample who could be located 8 months later, 20 had had a recurrence of the heart disease, and 7 had died as a direct consequence of the heart attack. The individuals who had had a recurrence of the disease, whether fatal or non-fatal, had reported significantly more worries at the first interview than people who had not suffered a recurrence. Somewhat similar findings were obtained in a large study reported by Ruberman *et al.* (1984). Thus, even though the evidence from retrospective studies of the impact of cumulative life stress on coronary heart disease is somewhat problematic, results from studies of the impact of bereavement and from prospective studies with high-risk groups provide consistent evidence on the relationship between psychosocial stress and heart disease.

Summary and conclusions

The stress concept was made popular by Selye's work on the bodily responses of organisms exposed to stressors such as intensive heat or cold, non-lethal injections of toxic substances and infections. Selye suggested that these bodily reactions to stress were non-specific and helped the organism to cope with the stressor. Diseases of adaptation characteristic of the stage of exhaustion are the price the organism has to pay for the defense against extended exposure to stressor agents.

The psychosocial approach to stress is based on the assumption that psychosocial stress results in the same kind of bodily changes which Selye observed as a consequence of tissue damage. In this tradition, evidence was generated to demonstrate that specific life-events or cumulative life stress are associated with an increased risk of morbidity or even mortality.

This research related stressful life-events to the incidence of illness, but did not ask the question why certain psychological experiences are stressful and how the organism distinguishes stressful from positive events. This issue was later addressed by psychological theories of stress which analyze the cognitive processes that mediate between life-events and stress. Two approaches were described, the cognitive stress theory of Lazarus and the theory of learned helplessness of Seligman. Both theories conceive of stress as resulting whenever events are appraised as potentially harmful and when individuals perceive their resources to be insufficient to prevent the aversive outcome.

The last section of the chapter addressed the question of how stressful events can be detrimental to psychological and physical health. The impact of psychosocial stress is mediated by two pathways, a direct route via the body's physiology and an indirect route, affecting health through the person's behavior. The joint impact of these reactions to stress contributes to the development of ill health either by interacting with other causes of disease or by affecting the body's ability to resist.

Suggestions for further reading

Cohen, S. and Williamson, G.M. (1991). Stress and infectious disease in humans. *Psychological Bulletin*, 109, 5–24. Comprehensive review of research on the relationship between stress and infectious disease in humans.

Lazarus, R.S. and Folkman, S. (1984). *Stress, appraisal, and coping.* New York: Springer. In this classic monograph the authors review the literature on stress as it relates to the cognitive stress theory of Lazarus and his co-workers.

Peterson, C., Seligman, M.E.P. and Vaillant, G.E. (1988). Pessimistic explanatory style is a risk factor for physical illness: A thirty-five-year longitudinal study. *Journal of Personality and Social Psychology*, 55, 23–7. An interesting study testing predictions from the theory of learned helplessness. Attributional style assessed from interviews completed at age 25 years by Harvard graduates was found to be related to their health 20 to 35 years later.

Stroebe, M., Stroebe, W. and Hansson, R. (Eds) (1993). *Handbook of bereavement.* New York: Cambridge University Press. This edited volume provides a comprehensive review of scientific knowledge on the psychological and psychobiological consequences of losing a loved person through death.

Watson, D. and Pennebaker, J.W. (1989). Health complaints, stress, and distress: Exploring the central role of negative affectivity. *Psychological Review*, 96, 234–54. Argues that self-report measures of both stressful life events and health complaints reflect a pervasive mood disposition to experience negative mood. While negative affectivity correlates highly with measures of symptom reporting, it seems to be unrelated to objective health indicators.

MODERATORS OF THE STRESS–HEALTH RELATIONSHIP

When we interviewed a sample of bereaved individuals to assess the health consequences of the loss experience, we were impressed by the tremendous differences in the way these people coped with the event, differences that were often quite unrelated to situational indicators of the severity of the event (e.g. Stroebe *et al.* 1988). Such differences in adjustment are naturally consistent with the inter-actional concept of stress, according to which individual differences in coping styles and coping resources are as important as variations in situational demands in determining the extent to which stress is experienced. This section will present a more detailed discussion of coping processes and of the major coping resources which moderate the relationship between stress and ill health.

Strategies of coping

Coping strategies or styles play an important role in an individual's physical and psychological well-being when he or she is confronted with negative or stressful life-events (Endler and Parker 1990). Recent research considers coping as "the person's cognitive and behavioral efforts to manage (reduce, minimize, master, or tolerate) the internal and external demands of the person–environment transaction that is appraised as taxing or exceeding the resources of the person" (Folkman *et al.* 1986b: 572). Thus coping encompasses the cognitive and behavioral strategies which individuals use both to manage a stressful situation and the negative emotional reactions elicited by that event.

The most striking feature of this definition of coping is its breadth. Thus, coping processes are not only assumed to include all the decisions and actions taken by an individual faced with a stressful life-event, but also the attendant negative emotions. The only limiting condition is that to constitute coping, these cognitive and behavioral strategies should have the function of "managing" the stressful situation. This implies that to constitute coping, strategies should *aim* at lowering the probability of harm resulting from the stressful encounter and/or at reducing negative emotional reactions. Whether these strategies are successful or not in reaching the goal of managing the stressful situation is not part of the definition of coping.

Dimensions of coping

A great deal of research effort has been invested in the identification of basic dimensions of coping. This is not surprising, since analyses of the literature on coping or of self-reports of cognitive or behavioral coping strategies employed by samples of respondents in stressful encounters have suggested an immense variety of coping strategies. In these investigations, respondents were presented with a list of coping strategies and asked to indicate which of these they used in coping with a recent stress experience. Their responses were then factor-analyzed. Factor analysis is a statistical procedure which allows one to identify from the intercorrelations of a list of items a smaller number of basic dimensions assumed to be responsible for these correlations.

The studies which followed this procedure uncovered a variety of different basic dimensions (e.g. Folkman and Lazarus 1980; Folkman et al. 1986a, 1986b; Amirkhan 1990; Endler and Parker 1990; Rohde et al. 1990). In a study which resulted in the construction of one of the most widely used coping scales, the Ways of Coping Questionnaire, Folkman et al. (1986a) identified eight distinct coping strategies (see Table 7.1). Endler and Parker (1990), on the other hand, who used a comparable procedure in the development of their Multidimensional Coping Inventory, arrived at three dimensions, namely task-oriented coping, emotion-oriented coping and avoidance-oriented coping. The factor-analytic study of Amirkhan (1990) also led to the distinction of three dimensions, but these were somewhat different from those identified by

Table 7.1 The coping strategies identified by Folkman and her colleagues

Scale 1: Confrontive coping	*Scale 5: Accepting responsibility*
Stood my ground and fought for what I wanted	Criticized or lectured myself
Tried to get the person responsible to change his or her mind	Realized I brought the problem on myself
I expressed anger to the person(s) who caused the problem	I made a promise to myself that things would be different next time
I let my feelings out somehow	
	Scale 6: Escape–avoidance
Scale 2: Distancing	Wished that the situation would go away or somehow be over with
Made light of the situation; refused to get too serious about it	Hoped a miracle would happen
Went on as if nothing had happened	Had fantasies about how things might turn out
Didn't let it get to me; refused to think about it too much	Tried to make myself feel better by eating, drinking, smoking, using drugs or medication, and so forth
Tried to forget the whole thing	
	Scale 7: Planful problem solving
Scale 3: Self-controlling	I knew what had to be done, so I doubled my efforts to make things work
I tried to keep my feelings to myself	I made a plan of action and followed it
Kept others from knowing how bad things were	Changed something so things would turn out all right
I tried to keep my feelings from interfering with other things too much	Drew on my past experiences; I was in a similar position before
	Scale 8: Positive reappraisal
Scale 4: Seeking social support	Changed or grew as a person in a good way
Talked to someone to find out more about the situation	I came out of the experience better than when I went in
Talked to someone who could do something concrete about the problem	Found new faith
I asked a relative or friend I respected for advice	Rediscovered what is important in life
Talked to someone about how I was feeling	

Source: Adapted from Folkman *et al.* (1986a).

Endler and Parker (1990). Amirkhan (1990) labelled his dimensions problem solving, seeking social support and avoidance.

There are a number of reasons for these inconsistencies. Far from being an objective procedure, the outcomes of factor analyses are dependent on numerous aspects of a study, such as the composition of the item pool or of the sample of respondents, and the method of factor analysis used. Finally, researchers have great freedom in the labels they attach to their scales, so that even apparent similarities between studies are often more the result of consistencies in labelling than in the items which underlie a dimension.

And yet it is possible to infer some consensus from these studies. There seem to be a number of basic dimensions which emerge in all of this research (for a review, see Parker and Endler 1992). Most studies suggest that coping has two major functions, namely to reduce the risk of harmful consequences that might result from a stressful event (i.e. problem-focused coping) and to regulate the distressing emotional reactions to the event (i.e. emotion-focused coping). While problem-focused coping is usually reflected by one or two factors, there is often a wide array of emotion-focused factors. Thus, two of the strategies identified by Folkman *et al.* (1986a) appear to be clearly problem-focused (confrontive coping, planful problem solving), five clearly emotion-focused (distancing, self-controlling, accepting responsibility, positive reappraisal) and one focusing on both functions (seeking social support).

A second dimension which frequently emerges from this research is approach *vs* avoidance. Avoidance coping is related to several constructs with a long research history (e.g. repression–sensitization, Byrne 1961; monitoring *vs* blunting, Miller 1980). An individual can confront his or her emotions (e.g. by reappraising the situation or confiding to a friend), but he or she can also avoid this confrontation by engaging in distracting activities (e.g. seeing a movie, visiting a friend). Similarly, an individual can confront a health threat by undergoing a recommended operation, but he or she might also decide that it would be better to avoid the operation. The Ways of Coping dimensions of distancing and escape–avoidance reflect avoidance strategies, whereas confrontive coping, accepting responsibility and planful problem solving would seem to involve approach-based coping.

A third dimension which has typically emerged in these studies is the seeking of social support. Individuals might cope with a stressful experience alone or seek social support to help reduce the

stress. As social psychologists, we would naturally like to add this
social dimension to coping. However, Endler and Parker (1990)
were probably right when they argued that social support should
be considered a resource for coping strategies rather than a specific coping dimension.

The differential effectiveness of strategies of coping

In view of the extensive research devoted to the identification of
basic dimensions of coping, it is surprising how little is known
about the differential effectiveness of these coping strategies. Even
though numerous studies have related coping strategies to physical
and psychological well-being following stressful encounters, few
general conclusions can be drawn from this research (some of
these will be reviewed later in our discussion of research on optimism). There are a number of theoretical and methodological
reasons for the failure of this outcome research to produce clear-
cut findings. Much of this work has been stimulated by the
interactional stress theory of Lazarus and his colleagues, a theory
which does not allow any predictions about the choice of coping
strategies or effectiveness of coping. There were also a number of
methodological weaknesses. First, most of the existing coping scales
suffer from psychometric problems (Endler and Parker 1990). Second, measures of coping assess only whether an individual used a
particular coping strategy but do not evaluate coping efficacy
(Aldwin and Revenson 1987). Thus, respondents may be asked to
what extent they conceived and followed a plan, but not whether
the plan was well designed or was carried out successfully. Third,
and in our view most importantly, research frequently assesses
coping effectiveness in relation to a range of *different* stressful
encounters. Typically, subjects are asked to indicate the most stressful event they experienced during a specified period, which may be
financial problems, health problems, interpersonal disputes or difficulties at work (e.g. Folkman *et al.* 1986b; McCrae and Costa
1986; Aldwin and Revenson 1987). In view of the general consensus in the literature that the effectiveness of a given coping
strategy is dependent on the nature of the stressful encounter, the
decision to adopt a procedure which aggregates measures of coping effectiveness across different encounters is surprising.

The one consistency which tends to emerge from this research is that, although avoidance coping strategies such as denial may be quite effective at certain times, for example early on in coping with traumatic events (see Stroebe 1992), the chronic use of avoidance coping strategies may be a risk factor for adverse responses to stressful life-events (e.g. Rohde *et al.* 1990; Carver *et al.* 1993; Stanton and Snider 1993). These findings are consistent with research by Pennebaker on the positive health impact of disclosure of previously undisclosed traumatic events. Pennebaker consistently found that subjects who had been instructed to write about past traumatic events (e.g. Pennebaker and Beall 1986; Pennebaker *et al.* 1988) or recent upsetting experiences (Pennebaker *et al.* 1990) reported fewer health center visits following the experiment when compared with controls who wrote about trivial events.

Pennebaker accounts for these findings in terms of his theory of inhibition, which outlines the processes by which failure to confront traumatic events results in poorer health. The central assumption of this theory is that inhibition of thoughts, feelings and behavior is an active process requiring physiological work. When individuals inhibit their desire to talk or think about traumatic experiences over long periods of time, cumulative stress is placed on the body resulting in increased vulnerability to stress-related disease. Thus, Pennebaker's findings might suggest one of the mechanisms mediating the health-impairing effect of chronic avoidance.

Coping resources as moderators of the stress–health relationship

According to cognitive stress theories, the impact of stress on health is also dependent on the coping resources which are available to the individual confronted with the stressful life-event. In analyzing coping resources, researchers distinguish between intrapersonal and extrapersonal resources (e.g. Lazarus and Folkman 1984; Stroebe and Stroebe 1987; Cohen and Edwards 1989). *Intrapersonal resources* consist of the personality traits, abilities and skills which enable persons to cope with the stress experience. The major *extrapersonal resources* are financial resources and social support, both of which are resources external to the individual and potentially helpful in alleviating the stress. Coping resources are sometimes referred to as "stress-buffering resources" because they are presumed to protect or buffer people from the negative impact of stressful events (e.g. Cohen and Edwards 1989).

Coping resources can moderate the impact of stressful life-events by influencing stress appraisal or by affecting the coping process (Cohen and Wills 1985). Most resources intervene at both of these stages. For example, the pessimistic attribution style conceptualized as part of the revised model of learned helplessness is assumed to moderate both appraisal and recovery (e.g. Peterson and Seligman 1987). Similarly, the extent to which individuals perceive supportive others as available will affect the appraisal as well as the coping process (Cohen and Wills 1985). Much of the empirical research on coping resources has investigated whether a person's health status is related to the extent to which he or she possesses a given resource. For example, as we see later, there is evidence that individuals who have a great deal of social support suffer a lower risk of mental and physical impairment and even mortality than individuals who have little social support.

Intrapersonal coping resources

Numerous personality variables have been suggested as moderators of the impact of stress on health, and the list of variables is continuously being extended. Since it would be too ambitious in the context of this chapter to attempt an exhaustive review of this rich but complex body of literature, we will restrict our presentation here to two personality variables that have been specifically developed and extensively studied in a health context – hardiness (e.g. Kobasa *et al.* 1982a) and dispositional optimism (e.g. Scheier and Carver 1987).

The hardy personality

Hardiness has been proposed by Kobasa (1979) as a constellation of personality characteristics that protect individuals against the health-impairing impact of stress. There are three components of the hardy personality: (1) *control*, which refers to people's belief that they can influence events in their lives; (2) *commitment*, which refers to people's sense of purpose and involvement in the events, activities and others in their lives; and (3) *challenge*, which refers to the expectation that change rather than stability is normal in life and that change in the form of life-events can be a positive phenomenon with the opportunity for growth, rather than a threat to security. Hardy individuals would score high on all three dimensions and would thus possess a life philosophy which buffers them against the debilitating impact of stressful life-events.

The measurement of hardiness

In the course of the development of the concept of hardiness, the scales used to measure it have changed. The most frequently used instrument to measure hardiness in recent research seems to be a composite of five scales: *control* is measured by the Powerlessness Scale of the Alienation Test (Maddi *et al.* 1979) and the External Locus of Control Scale (Rotter *et al.* 1962); *commitment* is measured by the Alienation from Self Scale and the Alienation from Work Scale of the Alienation Test (Maddi *et al.* 1979); *challenge* is measured by the Security Scale of the California Life Goals Evaluation Schedule (Hahn 1966). For each of these scales, a high score reflects a relative lack of hardiness.

The practice of combining the various scales used to measure hardiness into one overall score is based on the assumption that individual differences on these measures reflect a common dimension of hardiness. If this assumption is correct, correlations between individual scores on pairs of scales should be high and factor analyses of the five scales should yield a single factor. These assumptions have been questioned (e.g. Funk and Houston 1987; Hull *et al.* 1987; Cohen and Edwards 1989). In fact, Kobasa *et al.* (1981) report surprisingly low correlations between pairs of scales used to measure hardiness.

Hardiness and health

The concept of hardiness was developed and tested in a study which tried to differentiate people who reacted to stress with illness from those who stayed healthy on the basis of their personality. In a retrospective study, Kobasa (1979) selected from a sample of male executives of a large public utility company those who, in response to her questionnaire, reported high levels of stress for the previous 3 years on the Social Readjustment Rating Scale (Holmes and Rahe 1967). This high-stress group was divided into a high- and a low-illness group on the basis of their responses to a self-report checklist of more than 100 commonly recognized physical and mental illnesses and symptoms. The two groups were then sent a package of personality tests containing five personality scales for each component of the hardiness construct. Statistical analyses identified a number of scales that showed significant differences between the two groups. Kobasa (1979) interpreted these findings as support for her hypothesis that high-stress/low-illness executives indeed show more hardiness than high-stress/high-illness executives. However, although these findings are suggestive, they do not really demonstrate a buffering (i.e. protective) effect of hardiness. They might merely reflect a correlation between the scales used to measure hardiness and the self-report health measure. To rule out this interpretation and demonstrate buffering, Kobasa would have had to show that hardiness was unrelated (or at least substantially less related) to health in a low-stress group.

In two subsequent articles, Kobasa and her colleagues reported a buffering effect for hardiness in a retrospective study that used an adequate design (Kobasa et al. 1982b; Kobasa and Puccetti 1983). Kobasa and her colleagues also conducted a prospective study on executives of the same utility company, in which they collected three sets of data at 1 year intervals (Kobasa et al. 1981, 1982a). Using reported illness summed over years 2 and 3 as the dependent variable and year 1 stressful events, hardiness and constitutional predisposition (a measure of parents' illness) as predictors, they found significant main effects for stressful life-events, hardiness and constitutional predisposition. Although the pattern of means was consistent with a buffering effect for hardiness, no interactions were significant. However, Kobasa et al. (1982a) reported an analysis of the same data set which, controlling for illness at year 1 and dropping constitutional predisposition from the analysis, revealed a significant buffering effect.

Further evidence for a buffering effect of hardiness comes from a retrospective study of a sample of female former students of a small liberal arts college (Rhodewalt and Zone 1989). Life stress was measured with an adapted form of the Schedule of Recent Life Events. Subjects had to indicate which of the events they had experienced during the previous 12 months. They also had to rate whether the event was desirable or undesirable, controllable or uncontrollable, and the amount of adjustment that was necessary for them to cope with the event. Health was assessed with the Beck Depression Inventory (a self-report scale of common symptoms of depression) and the same illness rating scale used by Kobasa (1979). The authors found a buffering effect of hardiness for both depression and self-reported physical illness (Figure 7.1). Thus,

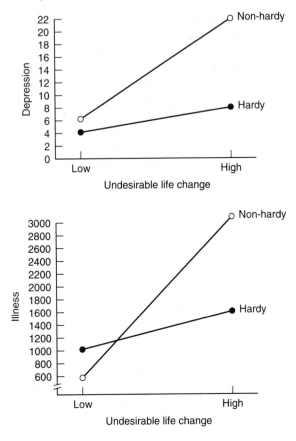

Figure 7.1 Predicted values of depression and illness for the
interaction of hardiness with undesirable life change
Source: Rhodewalt and Zone (1989)

hardiness seemed to protect these women somewhat against the
negative impact of stress on psychological and physical health.

This study is particularly interesting because it also assessed
hardiness-related differences in appraisal of stress. Although hardy
and non-hardy women did not differ in the absolute number of
stressful events reported, non-hardy women reported significantly
greater numbers of undesirable life changes. Thus, non-hardy
women declared that roughly 40 per cent of their life experiences
were undesirable, whereas their hardy counterparts appraised only

27 per cent of their experiences in this manner. In addition to appraising a greater number of events as negative, non-hardy women also reported that the negative events required more adjustment than did hardy women. These findings suggest that the buffering effect of hardiness is at least partly mediated by differences in appraisal processes.

However, there are also several studies which failed to find any evidence for a buffering effect (e.g. Schmied and Lawler 1986; Funk and Houston 1987); or observed buffering effects only for one of the components of the Hardiness Scale (e.g. Ganellen and Blaney 1984). Furthermore, there is evidence that hardiness is highly correlated with negative affectivity or neuroticism (Funk and Houston 1987; Hull *et al.* 1987; Allred and Smith 1989). As Watson and Pennebaker (1989) have shown, self-report measures of both stress and of health complaints reflect a pervasive mood disposition of negative affectivity or neuroticism. Thus, it may not be the hardy individuals who are particularly stress-resistant, but the non-hardy individuals who are neurotic and psychologically maladjusted and who therefore view their lives as more negative and stressful and also report higher levels of health complaints. As the findings of Watson and Pennebaker further suggest, these complaints could be *unrelated* to physical health problems. It would therefore be important in further studies to test whether the buffering effect of hardiness can be replicated with objective stress situations using biological or other objective indicators of health status.

Conclusions

There is suggestive evidence that hardiness protects individuals against the impact of stressful life-events and that this buffering effect is mediated by related differences in appraisal processes. Hardy individuals appear to view their lives more positively and as more under their own control. However, the fact that buffering studies have assessed both stress and health with self-report methodology is problematic, particularly in view of the high negative correlation between hardiness and neuroticism. Because of this, it remains unclear whether the observed interactions between hardiness and stress on health measures should be interpreted in terms of a protective effect of hardiness on health, or in terms of differences in the way neurotic individuals perceive and/or report stress and health symptoms.

Dispositional optimism

Dispositional optimism is a second personality variable which has recently been suggested as a moderator of the stress–health relationship. It has been proposed that an optimistic nature can motivate people to cope more effectively with stress and consequently reduce the risk of illness (Scheier and Carver 1987). The crucial factor in optimism, according to Scheier and Carver, is that optimists will be more likely to see desired outcomes as within their reach than pessimists. People who see desired outcomes as attainable should continue to exert effort to reach these outcomes, even if it is difficult. On the other hand, when outcomes are sufficiently unattainable people will reduce their efforts and eventually abandon the pursuit of a given goal.

Scheier and Carver began their research by developing a measure of dispositional optimism, the Life Orientation Test (LOT). The LOT is assumed to measure the extent to which individuals hold the general expectation that good things are likely to happen to them. The LOT consists of eight items, four phrased in a positive way (e.g. "In uncertain times, I usually expect the best") and four phrased in a negative way (e.g. "If something can go wrong for me, it will"), plus four irrelevant items used to distract respondents from the purpose of the scale. Respondents answer each item by indicating the extent of their agreement on a 5-point scale.

There is empirical evidence that individuals who score high on optimism suffer fewer symptoms of distress following stressful life-experiences than individuals with low optimism scores. In a study with undergraduates conducted during an examination period, optimism assessed at the beginning of the study was related to symptoms reported at the end of the study. Students who scored high on the optimism scale reported fewer physical symptoms 4 weeks later than students who scored low, and this relationship persisted even after investigators controlled for initial differences in symptom levels.

Scheier and Carver assume that the greater stress resistance of optimists is mediated by differences in coping strategies. Evidence for optimism-related differences in coping comes from a study by Scheier et al. (1986), who administered both the LOT and the Ways of Coping Questionnaire to a sample of undergraduates. Scheier et al. found that optimism was associated with a greater use of problem-focused coping, seeking of social support, and emphasizing the positive aspects of a stressful situation. In contrast, pessimism was associated with denial and distancing, and with focusing on the goal with which the stressor was interfering.

That the impact of optimism on differences in adjustment to the stresses of college life is indeed mediated by differences in coping styles has been demonstrated in a longitudinal study of college students who were interviewed twice, shortly after entering college and 3 months later (Aspinwall and Taylor 1992). Aspinwall and Taylor found that optimists made less use of avoidance coping. Avoidance coping in turn predicted less successful adjustment to college life 3 months later. Greater optimism was also related to the greater use of active coping. This in turn predicted better adjustment to college.

That optimism was an important predictor of coping efforts and of recovery from surgery was shown in a study of coronary bypass patients (Scheier et al. 1989). Optimists used more problem-focused coping and made less use of denial. They recovered faster from the effects of surgery and there was also a positive relationship between optimism and post-surgical quality of life 6 months later, with optimists doing substantially better than pessimists. Comparable findings were reported from a longitudinal study of women with early stage breast cancer. These women were interviewed before surgery and several times after surgery. Optimists reported less distress at each point of measurement than pessimists and this effect was mediated by aspects of the subjects' coping reactions, particularly the tendency of optimists to make less use of denial and behavioral disengagement.

However, like hardiness research, the research based on the optimism scale has been criticized for its overlap with negative affectivity and neuroticism (Smith et al. 1989). In a replication of the study of Scheier and Carver (1985) on undergraduate stress, Smith et al. administered a measure of negative affectivity in addition to the LOT. Their findings for the LOT were comparable to those reported by Scheier and Carver (1985) – optimists tended to engage more in problem-focused coping and less in avoidance coping than pessimists and they also reported fewer symptoms at the second assessment. However, these relationships disappeared when the level of neuroticism was statistically controlled. In contrast, the statistical control of optimism scores did not eliminate the relationship between neuroticism and these same symptoms. As Smith and colleagues (1989: 645) concluded: "at the very least, these findings suggest that optimism as defined by the LOT is not related to coping and symptom report independently of the influence of neuroticism".

Extrapersonal coping resources

Two major extrapersonal coping resources are material resources and social support. Whereas there is an extensive literature on social support as a coping resource (for reviews, see House 1981; Cohen and Wills 1985), economic resources are rarely discussed in this context (Lazarus and Folkman 1984). We will therefore consider the role of economic resources only briefly and devote most of this section to the discussion of the impact of social support on health and well-being.

Material resources

In view of the strong negative relationship which has been observed between social class and illness or social class and mortality, it is surprising that material resources are so infrequently discussed as a coping resource. It would seem plausible that the coping function of economic resources contributes to the negative association between socioeconomic status and morbidity or mortality. After all, people with money, especially if they have the skills to use it effectively, should have more coping options in most stressful situations than people without money. Money can provide easier access to legal, medical and other professional assistance.

The problem in using data on the association between socioeconomic status and health as evidence in this context is that the relationship itself is not very well understood. However, one of the major causes assumed to be responsible for the higher morbidity and mortality associated with low socioeconomic status has been exposure to stressful life-events. Moderate but significant positive correlations between socioeconomic status and life change scores indicate that stressful life-events are over-represented in the lower classes (e.g. Dohrenwend 1973). There is also evidence that exposure to undesirable life-events is more likely to evoke mental health problems in low rather than high socioeconomic status individuals (e.g. Dohrenwend 1973). The greater vulnerability of lower-class individuals seems to some extent to be due to a differential availability of social support (cf. Brown and Harris 1978). However, it is plausible that restricted access to other coping resources due to limited economic means could also contribute to this relationship.

If economic resources form an important coping resource, they should buffer the individual against the deleterious impact of stress. However, at least in bereavement research, the one area in which socioeconomic status has been studied as a stress moderator, there does not seem to be any evidence that high socioeconomic status buffers individuals against the health-impairing impact of the loss experience. While most studies show that the widowed of low socioeconomic status are less healthy than the widowed of high socioeconomic status, the comparison with non-bereaved control groups indicates that the health differential due to socioeconomic status is the same for bereaved and non-bereaved individuals (for a review, see Stroebe and Stroebe 1987). Clearly, though, the fact that economic resources do not appear to buffer the individual against the health impact of bereavement does not preclude the possibility that such resources could protect against other types of stressful events.

Social support

Over the past few decades, much research effort has been invested in the examination of the beneficial effects of social support on health and well-being. There is now a great deal of evidence that the availability of social support is associated with a reduced risk of mental illness and physical illness, and even mortality (e.g. Cohen and Wills 1985; Cohen 1988; House et al. 1988; Schwarzer and Leppin 1989a, 1989b). Social support has been defined as information from others that one is loved and cared for, esteemed and valued, and part of a network of communication and mutual obligation (Cobb 1976). Such information can come from a spouse, a lover, children, friends, or social and community contacts such as churches or clubs.

Conceptualization and measurement of social support
The measurement of social support has been approached from two perspectives, which differ in the way they conceptualize social

support. One conceives of social support in terms of the *structure* of the target person's interpersonal relationships or social network, the other in terms of the *functions* that these relationships or networks serve for him or her (for a discussion, see Cohen and Wills 1985; House and Kahn 1985).

Structural measures assess the existence or quantity of social relationships. This information is relatively objective and easy to obtain. It can sometimes be gathered by observation or from behavioral records (e.g. marriage records, organizational membership). But even if it is based on self-reports, information about whether a person is married, lives alone or belongs to some church is simple to collect, and usually fairly accurate (House and Kahn 1985). A standardized procedure for measuring various social network characteristics (e.g. size, density) has been developed by Stokes (1983) and is known as the Social Network List. There is consistent evidence that low levels of social relationship are associated with an increased risk of mortality (Berkman and Syme 1979; Blazer 1982; House *et al.* 1982).

Functional measures of social support assess whether interpersonal relationships serve particular functions. Various typologies of support functions have been proposed (e.g. House 1981; Cohen and McKay 1984; Stroebe and Stroebe 1987). Most distinguish between emotional, instrumental, informational and appraisal support. *Emotional support* involves providing empathy, care, love and trust. *Instrumental support* consists of behaviors that directly help the person in need; for example, individuals give instrumental support when they help other people to do their work, take care of their children or help them with transportation. *Informational support* involves providing people with information which they can use in coping with their problems. *Appraisal support* is closely related to informational support. It also involves the transmission of information, but in this case it is information that is relevant for the person's self-evaluation. Thus, by comparing oneself to another person, one may use the other as a source of information in evaluating oneself.

The measurement of social support functions has been based on measures assessing the individual's perception of either the availability of others who provide these functions or the actual receipt of these support functions during a given time period (for a discussion of this distinction, see Dunkel-Schetter and Bennett 1990). Examples of measures of the *perceived availability* of social support are the Interpersonal Support Evaluation List (ISEL: Cohen *et al.* 1985) and the Social Support Questionnaire (SSQ: Sarason *et al.* 1983). The ISEL assesses the perceived availability of four types of social support (tangible, appraisal, self-esteem, belonging). For example, respondents have to indicate whether there are people to whom they can talk about intimate personal problems or who would help them with advice. The items of the SSQ consist of two parts, one assessing the number of available others whom individuals feel they can "count on" for a particular type of support, and another measuring the individual's degree of satisfaction with the perceived support available in that particular situation. The number of available support providers is more similar to structural measures of social network size than to measures of functional support, and is only moderately related to the satisfaction with the social support that is available.

A widely used scale to assess *received* social support is the Inventory of Socially Supportive Behaviors (ISSB: Barrera *et al.* 1981). The items of the ISSB describe specific supportive behaviors that represent emotional, tangible, cognitive-informational and direct guidance support. Respondents are asked to indicate how often during the previous 4 weeks each supportive behavior occurred. The individual's score thus represents the average frequency of receipt of these supportive behaviors.

Relationships between measures

It would seem plausible that the number of social relationships a person has established is strongly related to the functional support the person perceives as available or actually receives. However, the different types of measures of social support show only weak relationships with each other. For example, Sarason *et al.* (1987), who examined the relationship between the Social Network List and measures of perceived and received social support (SSQ, ISSB), found only modest correlations between network size and satisfaction with perceived or received social support. These findings are reasonable if one considers that adequate functional support might be derived from *one* very good relationship but may not be available from many superficial ones.

The relationship between measures of the perceived availability of social support and received social support is also typically very modest. That low correlations are quite typical can be seen from Dunkel-Schetter and Bennett's (1990) survey of studies of the relationship between these two types of measures. These authors discuss a number of reasons why perceptions of availability of support should not be expected to be accurate reflections of the actual support one is likely to receive in situations of need.

A serious problem with measures of received social support is that the supportive behavior of others is not only a function of who is available but also of the instances in which help might have been needed during the period in question. It is therefore not surprising, that unlike measures of the perceived availability of support, measures of received support have often been found to be positively related to negative life-events and symptomatology (cf. Sarason *et al.* 1990).

Mediators of the relationship between social support and health

There are a number of psychological and biological processes through which social support might influence an individual's health. For example, a person who is integrated into a large social network of family and friends is subject to social controls and peer pressures that influence normative health behaviors. Depending on whether these pressures promote healthy or unhealthy behavior patterns, social integration could have a positive or negative impact on health (Cohen 1988). There is some evidence, however, that social support is positively associated with behaviors that are promotive of health (e.g. adherence to medical regimens or traditional health behaviors such as non-smoking, adequate sleep, prudent diet and moderate drinking behavior). Thus Berkman and Syme (1979) reported a positive relationship between their structural measure of support and various health practices. The possibility that social networks and social support influence health behaviors is also suggested by recent research on giving up smoking. These studies suggest that success in stopping smoking and the ability to maintain abstinence over a longer period of time has been linked to supportive behaviors from spouses and friends (for a review, see Cohen 1988).

Many of the *psychological* processes that link social support to psychological well-being and health may be mediated by self-esteem, that is, the positive or negative beliefs and evaluations that the individual holds towards him or herself. It is widely accepted among clinical, personality and social psychologists that a positive and stable self-esteem is important for individual well-being (e.g.

Epstein 1973). As Tajfel (1978, pp. 61–76) emphasized, the social groups to which we belong are major determinants of our definition of "self" and form the basis of social identity. Social identity refers to that part of people's self-concepts which derives from their knowledge of their memberships of various social groups, together with the emotional significance attached to these memberships. Thus, embeddedness in a large interpersonal and social network may contribute positively to social identity and self-esteem.

Social relationships may also fulfill a number of support functions which are beneficial for individual self-esteem. Thus, there is broad agreement among the helping professions concerning the central role of emotional support for self-esteem and psychological well-being. As Bernard (1968: 137) has described so graphically:

> One of the major functions of positive, expressive talk is to raise the status of the other, to give help, to reward; in ordinary human relations it performs the stroking function. As infants need physical caressing or stroking in order to live and grow, and even to survive, so do adults need emotional or psychological stroking or caressing to remain normal.

Group members also serve validational functions which are important for an individual's interpretation of reality. Success or failure in responding to situational demands depends not merely on one's skills but also on whether one is able to assess these abilities and the environmental demands realistically. Thus, people often fail because they overestimate their ability or underestimate the difficulty of the task. According to Festinger (1954), the assessment of the validity of one's beliefs about "reality" and about one's own level of ability frequently depend on social comparison processes, particularly when objective criteria are lacking. Social comparison processes are also important for the evaluation of the appropriateness of one's emotional reactions, particularly in novel, emotion-arousing situations (Schachter 1959). Such processes are therefore likely to play an important role in the perception and evaluation of bodily symptoms.

Ultimately, the impact of social and psychological variables on physical health must be transmitted through *biological* processes. In his classic book *The Broken Heart*, Lynch (1970) reported a variety of studies of animals and humans which suggest that the mere presence of, and especially affectionate physical contact with, another similar non-threatening organism can markedly reduce cardiovascular and other forms of physiological reactivity. There is also evidence that social support influences the neuroendocrine responses which have been suggested as possible mediators of the relationships between social support and coronary heart disease and between social support and immune functioning (for a review, see Cohen 1988). Suggestive evidence of a link between social support and immune function comes from studies showing that individuals with high scores on a loneliness scale exhibited some suppression of the immune system when compared with individuals who scored low on this scale (Kiecolt-Glaser *et al.* 1984; Glaser *et al.* 1985). Since loneliness is negatively correlated with perceived social support, these findings tend to support the assumption that low levels of social support are associated with the impairment of immune functions.

The impact of social support on health

Much of the impetus for the work on social support and health came from the field of epidemiology. In an impressive early survey, Berkman and Syme (1979) were able to demonstrate an extreme effect on health, namely a relationship between social support and mortality. These investigators studied social and community ties among a random sample of 6928 women and men aged 30–69 years when first interviewed in 1965 in Alameda County, California. Each of the four types of social relationships that was assessed at that time (marriage, contacts with extended family and friends, church membership, membership of other organizations) independently predicted the rate of mortality over the succeeding 9 years. Individuals who were low on an overall "social network" index, which weighted the intimate ties more heavily, had approximately twice the mortality risk of individuals who were high on this index over the 9 year period.

Do these findings really show that the availability of social networks extends one's life-span? One obvious alternative explanation is that the relationship between networks and mortality could have been due to the fact that isolated people were ill at the time of the survey and unable to maintain their social contacts. However, this appeared not to be the case, because the social network index continued to predict mortality after health status at the time of the baseline survey was statistically controlled.

Berkman and Syme (1979) had to rely on self-reports of physical health, cigarette smoking, alcohol consumption, obesity and level of physical activity. Since self-report health measures are not the most reliable or valid indicator of a person's health status, it was important to replicate these findings with more objective indicators of health status. This was done in a large-scale prospective study which was part of the Tecumseh Cummunity Health Study (House *et al.* 1982). The sample consisted of 2754 men and women aged 39–69 years at the outset of the study in 1967. In addition to an assessment of several classes of social relationships and activities, a wide range of health indicators was biomedically measured (e.g. blood pressure, cholesterol, respiratory functions, electrocardiograms). Again, composite indices of these relationships were inversely related to mortality over the 10–12 year follow-up period, even after adjustment for initial health status. People with low levels of social relationship had approximately twice the mortality risk of those with high levels.

This basic pattern has been replicated in a more recent study in the USA (see Schoenbach *et al.* 1986). Of the American studies, only the Evans County study (Schoenbach *et al.* 1986) also provided data on Afro-Americans. Although the levels of mortality vary greatly across studies, the patterns of prospective association between social integration and mortality are remarkably similar. This can be seen from Figures 7.2. and 7.3, which show the age-adjusted mortality rates for males and females, respectively, from those five studies for which parallel data could be extracted (House *et al.* 1988).

Less dire consequences of the lack of social support have also been established. In their meta-analyses of more than 100 studies of the relationship between social support and health which appeared between 1976 and 1987, Schwarzer and Leppin (1989a, 1989b) found that social support was not only significantly related to mortality but also to self-report measures of health status, physiological reactivity (e.g. blood pressure, heart rate) and – most strongly – to depression. However, the population effect sizes, which reflect the strength of these relationships, were fairly modest, suggesting that social support on average accounted for 1–4 per cent of the variance in the health measures used in the studies.

Since levels of stress were not assessed in these studies, it is unclear whether these findings merely reflect a generalized beneficial effect of social support, independent of stress, or whether social support buffered individuals against the deleterious impact of stress. Both hypotheses are discussed in the literature. Figure

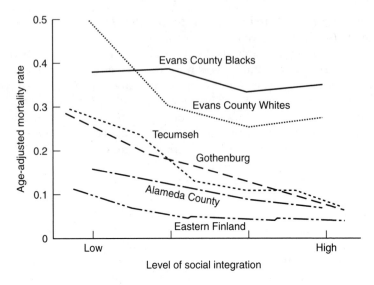

Figure 7.2 Level of social integration and age-adjusted mortality for males in five prospective studies
Source: Adapted from House *et al.* (1988)

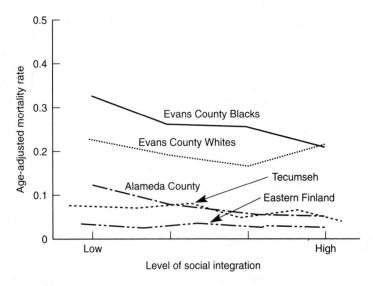

Figure 7.3 Level of social integration and age-adjusted mortality for females in five prospective studies
Source: Adapted from House *et al.* (1988)

Direct effect hypothesis

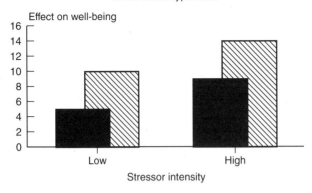

Buffering effect hypothesis

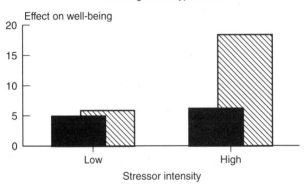

Figure 7.4 An illustration of the two ways in which social support is assumed to benefit health: the direct effect hypothesis proposes that the health benefits of social support occur irrespective of the level of stress; the buffering effect hypothesis proposes that social support protects individuals against the negative impact of high levels of stress. ■, high support; ▨, low support

7.4. illustrates the two ways in which social support can benefit health and well-being.

A *direct effect* of social support on health – independent of the amount of stress an individual experiences – could occur because large social networks provide people with regular positive experiences and a set of stable, socially rewarding roles in the community (Cohen and Wills 1985). For example, individuals with high levels of social support may have a greater feeling of being liked and cared for. The positive outlook this provides could be beneficial to health, independent of stress experience. A high level of social support may also encourage people to lead a more healthy lifestyle.

According to the *buffering hypothesis*, social support affects health by protecting the individual against the negative impact of high levels of stress (Figure 7.4). This protective effect can best be understood by means of an analogy with the effects of an inoculation. As a difference in the health of individuals who are or are not inoculated should emerge only when they are exposed to the infectious agent, the protective function of social support is effective only when the person encounters a strong stressor. Under low-stress conditions, little or no buffering occurs. Thus under low-stress conditions, no differences would be expected in the health and well-being of groups enjoying differential levels of social support.

Buffering could operate through two types of processes. First, individuals who enjoy a high level of social support may *appraise* a stressful event such as a financial crisis or the loss of a job as less stressful than people with little social support, because they know that there are people whom they can ask for advice or who would even be willing to support them financially. A second way in which social support might buffer the negative impact of stress is by improving people's ability to *cope* with the stressor. Thus, someone who is experiencing a crisis might be better able to cope if he or she knows people who can give advice or even provide a solution to the problem.

To differentiate between the direct effect and the buffering effect of social support, studies must assess the impact of differential levels of social support under differential levels of stress on health and well-being. The pattern that emerged from this type of research was less than clear-cut. Some studies reported only main effects, whereas others found interactions of stress and social support. In a review of this literature, Cohen and Wills (1985) examined the hypothesis that these differences in findings are related to the type of measure that was used in a given study. They reasoned that for a buffering effect to occur, the type of social support that is available should be closely linked to the specific coping needs elicited by a stressful event. Since only functional measures assess different types of social support, only studies using functional measures should yield buffering effects. The use of structural measures of social integration which only assess the existence or number of relationships, but not the functions actually provided by those relationships, should only result in main effects. Their review supported this hypothesis.

The role of personality dispositions in research on social support and health

A thorny issue that so far has not been addressed satisfactorily in research on social support and health is the possibility that personality dispositions could contribute to the observed relationship between measures of social support and health. There are two different routes by which personality could influence the relationship between social support and health. First, personality characteristics could increase an individual's chance of finding social support and at the same time contribute positively to his or her coping ability. For example, it seems plausible that individuals who are socially competent are also more likely to develop strong support networks and to stay healthy by effectively coping with stressful events or by performing health-enhancing behaviors (Cohen and Wills 1985). Second, personality characteristics might also bias individual reports of levels of social support and of health symptoms. This issue is particularly problematic where functional measures of social support and self-report measures of stress have been related to self-reports of psychological and physical symptoms. For example, in our Tübingen Study of Bereavement, a significant correlation (-0.32) was observed between a scale measuring perceived availability of social support and the Neuroticism Scale of the Eysenck Personality Inventory. Individuals who had high scores on neuroticism tended to report lower levels of perceived social support. Since, according to Watson and Pennebaker (1989), these individuals are also more likely to report higher levels of stressful life-events and higher levels of psychological and somatic symptoms, neuroticism could be partly responsible for relationships observed between measures of perceived social support, perceived stress and perceived symptomatology.

There are various strategies for dealing with these problems in research on perceived social support and health. One strategy is to reduce the influence of reporting biases by using objectifiable life-events (e.g. unemployment, bereavement) and biomedical health measures. A second safeguard is to use prospective designs which allow one to assess the impact of stress and social support measured at time 1 on symptomatology at time 2, while statistically controlling for differences in symptomatology at time 1. A third strategy involves the inclusion of measures of personality dispositions that are known correlates of social support (e.g. neuroticism, social competence) and using such measures as control variables.

The potential confounding influence of personality dispositions is less problematic in prospective epidemiological studies which relate measures of social integration to mortality. First, personality variables are less likely to influence the simple network measures typically used in these studies (e.g. reports about marriage, membership of organizations) than reports about the perceived availability of social support. Second, mortality is a dependent measure uninfluenced by this type of reporting bias. Finally, the alternative possibility that personality influences both the *actual* size of a person's social network (e.g. neurotics may be less likely to find partners or friends) and health can be controlled by using prospective designs that demonstrate the impact of social support on changes in health over time.

Summary and conclusions

This chapter has reviewed the impact of coping strategies and coping resources as moderators of the impact of stress on health. Research on basic dimensions of coping and on the differential effectiveness of coping strategies in alleviating the health-impairing impact of stress have led to few generalizable findings. The only consistency which tends to emerge is that avoidance coping strategies such as denial, distancing or escape, though probably sometimes effective in the early stages of coping with traumatic events, may be a risk factor for adverse responses to stressful events if used chronically.

We then reviewed research on personality characteristics and situational factors which serve as intrapersonal and extrapersonal coping resources and which help to protect individuals from the negative impact of stressful life-events. Our discussion of intrapersonal coping resources focused on two personality dimensions which have specifically been developed in the health context, the hardy personality and dispositional optimism. Hardiness consists of three components – control, commitment and challenge. It is believed that individuals who are high on these dimensions are better able to withstand the impact of stress and that this relationship is mediated by differences in appraisal processes. Hardy individuals are thought to evaluate stressful events as less stressful and threatening than non-hardy individuals. There is evidence for both the buffering effect of hardiness and for the mediating role of appraisal processes. However, due to the high correlation between hardiness and negative affectivity or neuroticism, it is somewhat unclear whether the buffering effect of hardiness should be interpreted in terms of a protective effect of hardiness on health, or in terms of differences in the way neurotic individuals perceive or report stress and health symptoms.

Perceived optimism was discussed as a second personality variable which is assumed to moderate the impact of stress on health and well-being. It has been assumed that the greater stress resistance of optimists is mediated by differences in coping strategies. In particular, optimists should be more likely to engage in problem-focused coping, while pessimists should use denial and distancing as preferred ways of coping. Evidence was presented to support this assumption. However, like hardiness, optimism is correlated with neuroticism and it is not yet clear to what extent neuroticism may be responsible for the relationship between optimism and health and well-being.

Our discussion of interpersonal coping resources focused mainly on the beneficial effect of social support on health and the role of social support as a stress-buffering resource. There is consistent evidence from epidemiological studies that individuals with low levels of social support are at greater risk of morbidity and mortality. There is also evidence that the perceived availability of social support buffers individuals against the impact of stressful life-events. Biological, behavioral and psychological processes were discussed which are assumed to mediate the positive impact of social support on health.

The body of research reviewed in this chapter has identified important personal and interpersonal resources which appear to protect individuals against the deleterious impact of stressful life-events, or might also help to reduce exposure to stressful situations. Since the impact on health of most intrapersonal resources seems to be mediated either by cognitive appraisal or by coping processes, this research raises the possibility that one could direct intervention toward the modification of styles of appraisal or coping. Furthermore, since both appraisal and coping are affected by social support, it might also be helpful to provide people with extrapersonal resources such as social support, and thereby improve their capacity to deal with stress.

Suggestions for further reading

Aspinwall, L.G. and Taylor, S.E. (1992). Modeling cognitive adaption: A longitudinal investigation of the impact of individual differences and coping on college adjustment and performance. Journal of Personality and Social Psychology, 63, 989–1003. Longitudinal study which suggests that differences in coping styles mediate the role of optimism as a moderator of the stress-health relationship.

Cohen, S. (1988). Psychosocial models of the role of social support in the etiology of physical disease. Health Psychology, 7, 269–97. A theoretical and empirical review of the mechanisms which mediate the relationship between social support and health.

Folkman, S., Lazarus, R.S., Dunkel-Schetter, C., Delongis, A. and Gruen, R. (1986). The dynamics of a stressful encounter. Journal of Personality and Social Psychology, 50, 992–1003. This study, in which the authors identified eight distinct coping strategies, resulted in the construction of the Ways of Coping Questionnaire, still one of the most widely used coping scales.

Funk, S.C. and Houston, B.K. (1987). A critical analysis of the hardiness scale's validity and utility. Journal of Personality and Social Psychology, 53, 572–8.

Sarason, B.R., Sarason, I.G. and Pierce, G.R. (Eds) (1990). Social support: An interactional view. New York: John Wiley. This edited volume contains chapters by many of the leading authorities on research on social support. It is currently the most comprehensive review of the field.

8 / THE ROLE OF SOCIAL PSYCHOLOGY IN HEALTH

The epidemiologic data presented in this book have identified health-impairing behavior patterns and psychosocial stress as important factors contributing to ill health. Social psychological knowledge can potentially be used to change health-impairing behavior patterns and to reduce psychosocial stress, thus enabling social psychologists to make a major contribution to the public health effort. In this last chapter, we would like to summarize our personal view on how social psychology should realize this potential.

Persuading people to change

A first important step in developing interventions aimed at changing health-impairing behavior patterns is the analysis of the psychological factors which determine this behavior and of the processes by which they operate. The social psychological models of behavior presented in Chapter 2 have identified factors such as attitudes toward a given behavior, subjective norms, and perceived control or self-efficacy as major determinants of behavior. The knowledge of the structure of beliefs and values underlying a given behavior pattern provides a scientific basis for the design of persuasive communications.

In developing persuasive communications to change attitudes and behavior, one would also rely on dual-process theories of attitude change (Chapter 3). These theories assume that the type of communication used in a campaign has to depend on the target audience's ability and motivation to scrutinize arguments. Only when an audience is sufficiently knowledgeable and motivated to assess the message and to match arguments to relevant pieces of knowledge, will the impact of the communication depend on the quality and forcefulness of the arguments contained in the communication. If, on the other hand, individuals are unwilling or unable to expend effort at processing arguments, they are likely to base their decision to accept or reject the message on some peripheral aspect such as the credibility or even attractiveness of the source of the communication. Thus, an analysis of the belief structure underlying a health-impairing behavior pattern may be most important when persuasive campaigns are directed at target audiences which are both motivated and able to scrutinize the arguments contained in a communication.

Limits to persuasion

Despite substantial developments in our understanding of the principles that underlie the formation and change of attitudes, the impact of programs of health education on health-impairing behavior patterns has often been disappointing. Attempts at persuading people to change their lifestyles have been hampered by two factors. First, it is difficult to convince people that they are vulnerable to a health risk and, second, even if individuals are persuaded to change health-impairing behaviors, they often find it difficult to act on these intentions.

As we discussed in Chapter 3, there is a discrepancy between individual and population perspectives of health risk. While public health policies are guided by the *population attributable risk* – that is, the number of excess cases of disease in a population that can be attributed to a given risk factor – individual decision making is determined by absolute and relative risk. The problem with many health-impairing behavior patterns is that the *relative risk* – that is, the ratio of chance of the disease for individuals who engage in a risky behavior and those who do not – is rather low. For example, even though drinking a bottle of wine every day or having a sedentary lifestyle increases the risk of morbidity and premature mortality, the relative risk is modest. And yet, because these habits are very common in Western societies, the excess burden on the population attributable to these risk factors is quite high.

But even if the relative risk attributable to a given behavior is high, the *absolute risk* may still be so low as to make it hardly seem worthwhile for the individual to change. For example, in the study of Harvard alumni (Paffenbarger *et al.* 1978) described earlier, sedentary men (i.e. index below 2000 kcal/week) ran twice the risk of suffering a fatal heart attack during the 6 to 10 year period of observation than their more active classmates. However, the fact that of the 16,936 Harvard alumni only 215 experienced fatal heart attacks during this period suggests that even with a sedentary life style the absolute risk was rather low. And yet these small numbers have a great significance from a *population perspective*, if one remembers that even in the USA only 15 per cent of the population exercise regularly in their leisure time (Oldridge 1984). Thus, thousands will die prematurely of a heart attack due to their lack of exercise. From the *perspective of the individual*, on the other hand, the odds are heavily in favor of individual survival, even without behavior change. An additional problem is that people's perceptions are often distorted by false optimism. They tend to believe that their personal risk is much lower than the relative risk for other people. For example, most car drivers rate themselves above average in their driving ability and smokers often feel that they are protected from ill health by a particularly hardy constitution.

Even if health education is effective in persuading people to change health-impairing lifestyles, people often fail to act according to their intentions. Thus, the chances of smokers stopping smoking at their first attempt is very low. Most people relapse within the first few months and need many repeated attempts before they succeed, if they succeed at all.

Some of these individuals can be helped by therapy. But despite recent improvements in methods of therapy, the painful fact which emerges from a review of the literature is that therapy, like medicine, has to be bitter to be helpful. The most striking demonstration of this fact is provided by research on the use of anorectic drugs in weight loss. Even though a combination of drug and behavior therapy resulted in much greater weight loss than behavior therapy alone, behavior therapy patients were much better able to maintain their weight loss than patients who had undergone the combined treatment (see Figure 4.5). It seems to be important that people attribute their weight loss to their ability to control their eating behavior. This perception of self-efficacy may not develop when weight loss can be attributed to the use of an anorectic drug.

Beyond persuasion: Changing the incentive structure

To some extent, these barriers can be circumvented by changing the rewards and costs associated with a given behavior. Thus, there is evidence that increases in the price of cigarettes or alcoholic beverages reduce the demand for these goods. Similarly, legal restrictions, like increasing the minimal age at which adolescents are allowed to purchase alcohol, or making seatbelt use compulsory, also have a positive impact on behavior. The advantage of legal and economic strategies is that they are useful for both influencing existing habits and preventing new health-impairing habits from developing.

However, there are also limits to the applicability of these strategies. Thus, economic incentives can only be employed in areas in which substances or goods have to be purchased to engage in certain health behaviors. And as the example of drug addiction demonstrates, high prices do not necessarily prevent people from abusive consumption. Similarly, legal sanctions can only be employed in areas where such sanctions are culturally acceptable and are also enforceable. For example, a law prescribing that condoms must always be used in sexual intercourse would be neither acceptable in our society, nor enforceable. The effectiveness of legal sanctions depends on the acceptance of the law and on individual perception that violation of the law is associated with a high risk of sanction. For example, it is quite likely that the introduction of a law making seatbelt use compulsory would not have been as effective as it was if people had not accepted that such a law was in their own best interest. In fact, without the persuasion campaign that made it widely known that the wearing of seatbelts substantially reduced the risk of injuries in traffic accidents, it is unlikely that such a law would have been introduced. Similarly, the significant increases in state taxes on cigarettes in the USA were only possible after extensive health education campaigns changed the public's perception of smoking. Thus, the war against smoking is an excellent example of the impact of a public health campaign that orchestrates persuasion with economic and legal means of changing health behavior.

Freedom and constraint

Thus, the data presented in this book tend to support the argument developed by Gary Becker (1976) that most deaths are to some extent self-inflicted in the sense that they could have been postponed if people had engaged in a healthy lifestyle or abandoned health-impairing behavior patterns. This has important implications both for individual decision making and public health policy. At the individual level, the implication is that people are free to choose between lifestyles which differ in their impact on their health. For example, it is up to the individual to decide whether he or she wants to smoke and risk premature death or stop the habit and thus reduce substantially the risk of morbidity and mortality from cancer and heart disease.

The important implication for public health policy is that it has to be ensured that the choices people make are well-informed ones. Individuals must be made to understand the health implications of their chosen lifestyle. But why should governments use legal measures and tax incentives to influence *individual* behavior and thus infringe on the freedom of their citizens to live according to their chosen lifestyles? After all, the days when suicide was a criminal offence in many countries are over. Accordingly, one could argue that people should be free to choose slow methods of suicide such as chain-smoking cigarettes or drinking too much alcohol.

However, there are reasons for governments to impose some constraint on individual freedom. One reason is that governments tend to discourage individual behavior which interferes with the health and well-being of others. Thus, the laws which forbid people to "drink and drive" are usually justified by the argument that drunken drivers are a danger to their fellow citizens and actually kill many of them every year. Similarly, passive smoking has now been recognized as a health risk. It has been estimated that in the UK, for example, approximately 1000 people die each year from passive smoking. According to one newspaper report, people who believe that their health was damaged in childhood by passive smoking have begun taking legal advice about sueing their parents (*Independent on Sunday*, January 31, 1993). This has led to the restrictions that have been imposed on smokers in airplanes, public buildings and offices.

But is there any justification to constrain people's freedom to choose behavior patterns that *impair only their own health*, such as imposing legal sanctions for a failure to wear seatbelts, or increasing taxes on cigarettes to reduce consumption? It has to be recognized that allowing individuals to impair their own health in this way also imposes a burden on their fellow citizens. Health, or more precisely the costs of illness, constitute a public good. Persons who supply or produce a public good cannot prevent those who do not contribute to it from consuming or benefiting from it. For example, clean air is a public good in the sense that people who incur costs or suffer discomfort to avoid contributing to pollution (e.g. by using public transport instead of their car) cannot prevent others, who do not incur such costs, from profiting from their actions. Thus, there is a temptation to free-ride. Similarly, health costs are a public good in countries in which there is full health insurance coverage, since contributions to insurance are usually independent of lifestyle factors. Thus, people who engage in health-impairing behavior patterns, and as a result incur higher health costs, free-ride to some extent on the healthful behavior of others.

Summary and implications

In this book, we have argued for integrated public health interventions that use both persuasion and incentives to influence a given behavior. Wherever feasible, environmental changes should also be introduced to reduce or eliminate the need for behavior change. For example, technical appliances should be constructed in ways that minimize the possibility of self-inflicted damage through careless operators. We would finally argue for a change in public health goals from quantity to quality of life. The substantial extension in life-expectancy during this century raised hopes that further improvements in medical treatment and healthy living would enable us to push the limits of mortality further and further. This hope has proved to be misplaced. There are strong indications that the rate at which the average life-expectancy increased during this century has declined sharply in the 1980s. The most favored populations, such as women who have already reached age 65, have a life-expectancy today which is exactly the same as it was in 1979 (Fries et al. 1989). Furthermore, physicians in the USA, who have modified risk factors well in advance of the general population and in directions reflecting the most recent knowledge (only 6 per cent of US physicians still smoke cigarettes), hardly live longer than their high-school classmates of the same race (Fries et al. 1989). We may have to accept the bitter truth that however far we jog, we will not live to be 140. Fortunately, there is more to life than the absence of death. Even though healthy living may not substantially extend our lifespan, it is likely to improve the quality of life and to extend *active* life-expectancy. By significantly reducing the average number of sick days, hospital days or illness symptoms, a healthy lifestyle will not only improve the quality of life for the individual, it will also result in a significant reduction in medical expenditure.

REFERENCES

Abel, E.L. (1980). Fetal alcohol syndrome: Behavioral teratology. *Psychological Bulletin*, 87, 29–50.

Abraham, S.C.S., Sheeran, P., Spears, R. and Abrams, D. (1992). Health beliefs and the promotion of HIV-preventive intentions among teenagers: A Scottish perspective. *Health Psychology*, 11, 363–70.

Abramson, L.Y., Seligman, M.E.P. and Teasdale, J.D. (1978). Learnt helplessness in humans: Critique and reformulation. *Journal of Abnormal Psychology*, 87, 49–74.

Adoph, E.F. (1947). Urges to eat and drink in rats. *American Journal of Physiology*, 151, 110–25.

Ajzen, I. (1988). *Attitudes, personality and behavior*. Chicago, IL: Dorsey Press.

Ajzen, I. (1991). The theory of planned behavior. *Organizational Behavior and Human Decision Processes*, 50, 179–211.

Ajzen, I. and Fishbein, M. (1975). *Belief, attitude, intention and behavior: An introduction to theory and research*. Reading, MA: Addison-Wesley.

Ajzen, I. and Fishbein, M. (1977). Attitude–behavior relations: A theoretical analysis and review of empirical research. *Psychological Bulletin*, 84, 888–918.

Ajzen, I. and Madden, T.J. (1986). Prediction of goal-directed behavior: Attitudes, intentions, and perceived behavioral control. *Journal of Experimental Social Psychology*, 22, 453–74.

Ajzen, I. and Timko, C. (1986). Correspondence between health attitudes and behavior. *Journal of Basic and Applied Psychology*, 42, 426–35.

Akiba, S., Kato, H. and Blot, W.J. (1986). Passive smoking and lung cancer among Japanese women. *Cancer Research*, 46, 4804–807.

Alcoholics Anonymous (1955). *The story of how many thousands of men and women have recovered from alcoholism*. New York: Alcoholics Anonymous Publishing.

Aldwin, C.M. and Revenson, T.A. (1987). Does coping help? A reexamination of the relation between coping and mental health. *Journal of Personality and Social Psychology*, 53, 337–48.

Allon, N. (1973). The stigma of overweight in everyday life. In G.A. Bray (Ed.), *Obesity in perspective*, Vol. 2, pp. 83–102. DHEW Publication No. (NIH) 75–708. Washington, DC: US Government Printing Office.

Allred, K.D. and Smith, T.W. (1989). The hardy personality: Cognitive and physiological responses to evaluative threat. *Journal of Personality and Social Psychology*, 56, 257–66.

American Cancer Society (1986). *Cancer, fact and figures*. New York: American Cancer Society.

American College of Sports Medicine Position Statement (1979). The recommended quantity and quality of exercise for developing and maintaining fitness in healthy adults. *Medicine and Science in Sports*, 10, 7–9.

American Psychiatric Association (1987). *Diagnostic and statistical manual of mental disorders. (DSM-III-R)*. Washington, DC: American Psychiatric Association.

Amirkhan, J.H. (1990). A factor analytically derived measure of coping: The coping strategy indicator. *Journal of Personality and Social Psychology*, 59, 1066–74.

Aral, O. (1993). Heterosexual transmission of HIV: The role of other sexually transmitted infections and behavior in its epidemiology, prevention and control. *Annual Review of Public Health*, 14, 451–67.

Aronson, E. and Carlsmith, J.M. (1963). Effect of severity of threat on the valuation of fobidden behavior. *Journal of Abnormal and Social Psychology*, 9, 233–71.

Ashley, M.J. and Rankin, J.G. (1988). A public health approach to the prevention of alcohol-related problems. *Annual Review of Public Health*, 9, 233–71.

Aspinwall, L.G. and Taylor, S.E. (1992). Modeling cognitive adaptation: A longitudinal investigation of the impact of individual differences and coping on college adjustment and performance. *Journal of Personality and Social Psychology*, 63, 989–1003.

Autorengruppe Nationales Forschungsprogramm (1984). *Wirksamkeit der Gemeindeorientierten Prävention Kardiovascularer Krankheiten (Effectiveness of community-oriented prevention of cardiovascular diseases)*. Bern: Hans Huber.

Avogaro, P. (1984). Apolipoproteins, the lipid hypothesis, and ischemic heart disease. In R.M. Kaplan and M.H. Criqui (Eds), *Behavioral epidemiology and disease prevention*, pp. 49–59. New York: Plenum Press.

Azrin, N.H. (1976). Improvements in the community-reinforcement approach to alcoholism. *Behaviour, Research and Therapy*, 6, 7–12.

Baer, J.S. and Lichtenstein, E. (1988). Classification and prediction of smoking relapse episodes: An exploration of individual differences. *Journal of Consulting and Clinical Psychology*, 56, 104–110.

Bahrke, M.S. and Morgan, W.P. (1978). Anxiety reduction following exercise and meditation. *Cognitive Therapy and Research*, 2, 323–33.

Bandura, A. (1986). *Social foundations of thought and action: A cognitive social theory*. Englewood Cliffs, NJ: Prentice-Hall.

Bandura, A., O'Leary, A., Taylor, C.B., Gauthier, J. and Gossard, D. (1987). Perceived self-efficacy and pain control: Opioid and nonopioid mechanisms. *Journal of Personality and Social Psychology*, 53, 563–71.

Barrera, M., Jr, Sandler, I.N. and Ramsey, T.B. (1981). Preliminary development of a scale of social support: Studies on college students. *American Journal of Community Psychology*, 9, 435–47.

Batchelor, W.F. (1988). AIDS 1988: The Science and the Limits of Science. American Psychologist, 43, 853–8.

Baucom, D.H. and Aiken, P.A. (1981). Effect of depressed mood on eating among obese and nonobese dieting persons. *Journal of Personality and Social Psychology*, 41, 577–585.

Beck, A.T. (1976). *Cognitive therapy and the emotional disorders*. New York: International Universities Press.

Becker, G.S. (1976). *The economic approach to human behavior*. Chicago, IL: University of Chicago Press.

Becker, M.H. and Joseph, J.G. (1988). AIDS and behavioral change to reduce risk: A review. *American Journal of Public Health*, 78, 394–410.

Beckman, H., Egbert, M.H., Post, R. and Goodwin, E.K. (1979). Effects of moderate exercise on Urinary MHPG in depressed patients. Pharmakopsychiatry, 12, 351–6.

Bellack, A.S. (1977). Behavioral treatment for obesity: Appraisal and recommendations. In M. Hersen, R.M. Eisler and P.M. Miller (Eds), *Progress in behavior modification*, pp. 1–38. New York: Academic Press.

Belloc, N.B. (1973). Relationship of health practices to mortality. *Preventive Medicine*, 2, 67–81.

Belloc, N.B. and Breslow, L. (1972). Relationship of physical health status and health practices. *Preventive Medicine*, 5, 409–421.

Bentler, P.M. and Speckart, G. (1979). Models of attitude–behavior relations. *Psychological Review*, 86, 452–64.

Bentler, P.M. and Speckart, G. (1981). Attitudes "cause" behaviors: A structural equation analysis. *Journal of Personality and Social Psychology*, 40, 226–38.

Berg, D., LaBerg, J.C., Skutte, A. and Ohman, A. (1981). Instructed versus pharmacological effects of alcohol in alcoholics and social drinkers. *Behavioral Research and Therapy*, 19, 55–66.

Berkman, L.F. and Syme, S.L. (1979). Social networks, host resistance, and mortality: A nine-year follow-up of Alameda County residents. *American Journal of Epidemiology*, 109, 186–204.

Bernard, J. (1968). *The sex game*. Englewood Cliffs, NJ: Prentice-Hall.

Best, J.A., Owen, L.E. and Trentadue, L. (1978). Comparison of satiation and rapid smoking in selfmanaged smoking cessation. *Addictive Behaviors*, 3, 71–8.

Best, J.A., Thompson, S.J., Santi, S.M., Smith, E.A. and Brown, K.S. (1988). Preventing cigarette-smoking among schoolchildren. *Annual Review of Public Health*, 9, 161–201.

Bigelow, G., Strickler, D., Liebson, I. and Griffiths, R. (1976). Maintaining disulfiram ingestion among outpatient alcoholics: A security deposit contingency contracting procedure. *Behavior Research and Therapy*, 14, 378–81.

Billman, G.E., Schwartz, P.J. and Stone, H.L. (1984). The effects of daily exercise on susceptibility to sudden cardiac death. *Circulation*, 69, 1182–9.

Björntorp, P. (1986). Fat cells and obesity. In K.D. Brownell and J.P. Foreyt (Eds), *Handbook of eating disorders*, pp. 88–98. New York: Basic Books.

Björntorp, P., Carlgren, G., Isaksson, B., Krotkievski, M., Larsson, B. and Sjöström, L. (1975). Effect of an energy-reduced dietary regimen in relation to adipose tissue cellularity in obese women. *American Journal of Clinical Nutrition*, 28, 445–52.

Blackburn, G.L., Lynch, M.E. and Wong, S.L. (1986). The very-low-calorie diet: A weight-reduction technique. In K.D. Brownell and J.P. Foreyt (Eds), *Handbook of eating disorders*, pp. 198–212. New York: Basic Books.

Blackburn, H. (1983). Diet and atherosclerosis: Epidemiologic evidence and public health implications. *Preventive Medicine*, 12, 2–10.

Blair, S.N., Kohl III, H.W., Paffenbarger, R.S., Jr, Clark, D.G., Cooper, K.H. and Gibbons, L.W. (1989). Physical fitness and all-cause mortality: A prospective study of healthy men and women. *Journal of the American Medical Association*, 3, 2395–401.

Blane, H.T. and Leonard, K.E. (Eds) (1987). *Psychological theories of drinking and alcoholism*. New York: Guilford Press.

Blazer, D.G. (1982). Social support and mortality in an elderly community population. *American Journal of Epidemiology*, 115, 684–94.

Bliss, R.E., Garvey, A.J., Heinold, J.W. and Hitchcock, J.L. (1989). The influence of situation and coping on relapse crisis outcomes after smoking cessation. *Journal of Consulting and Clinical Psychology*, 57, 443–9.

Bohman, M. (1978). Some genetic aspects of alcoholism and criminality: A population of adoptees. *Archives of General Psychiatry*, 35, 269–76.

Bohman, M., Sigvardsson, S. and Cloninger, C.R. (1981). Maternal inheritance of alcohol abuse. *Archives of General Psychiatry*, 38, 965–9.

Bosello, O., Ostuzzi, R., Rossi, F.A. *et al.* (1980). Adipose tissue cellularity and weight reduction forecasting. *American Journal of Clinical Nutrition*, 33, 776–82.

Boster, F.J. and Mongeau, P. (1984). Fear-arousing persuasive messages. In R.N. Bostrom (Ed.), *Communication yearbook*, Vol. 8, pp. 330–75. Beverly Hills, CA: Sage.

Bouchard, C. and Pérusse, L. (1993). Genetics of obesity. *Annual Review of Nutrition*, 13, 337–54.

Brand, R.J., Paffenbarger, R.S., Sholtz, R.I. and Kampert, J.B. (1979). Work activity and fatal heart attack studied by multiple logistic risk analysis. *American Journal of Epidemiology*, 110, 52–62.

Bray, G.A. (1986). Effects of obesity on health and happiness. In K.D. Brownell and J.P. Foreyt (Eds), *Handbook of eating disorders*, pp. 3–44. New York: Basic Books.

Breslow, L. and Enstrom, J.E. (1980). Persistence of health habits and their relationship to mortality. *Preventive Medicine*, 9, 469–83.

Brewin, C.R. (1988). *Cognitive foundations of clinical psychology*. Hove: Lawrence Erlbaum Associates Ltd.

Brooks, C.M., Marine, D.N. and Lambert, E.F. (1946). A study of the oxygen consumption of albino-rats during various phases of experimentally produced obesity. *American Journal of Physiology*, 147, 717–26.

Brown, G.W. and Harris, T. (1978). *Social origins of depression: A study of psychiatric disorder in women.* New York: Free Press.

Brownell, K.D. (1982). Obesity: Understanding and treating a serious, prevalent and refractory disorder. *Journal of Consulting and Clinical Psychology*, 50, 820–40.

Brownell, K.D. (1983). Assessment in the treatment of eating disorders. In D.H. Barlow (Ed.), *Behavioral assessment of adult disorders*, pp. 329–404. New York: Guilford Press.

Brownell, K.D. and Wadden, T.A. (1986). Behavior therapy for obesity: Modern approaches and better results. In K.D. Brownell and J.P. Foreyt (Eds), *Handbook of eating disorders*, pp. 180–97. New York: Basic Books.

Brownell, K.D., Stunkard, A.J. and Albaum, J.M. (1980). Evaluation and modification of exercise patterns in the natural environment. *American Journal of Psychiatry*, 137, 1540–45.

Brownell, K.D., Marlatt, G.A., Lichtenstein, E. and Wilson, G.T. (1986). Understanding and preventing relapse. *American Psychologist*, 41, 765–82.

Brunner, D., Manelis, G., Modan, M. and Levin, S. (1974). Physical activity at work and the incidence of myocardial infarction, angina pectoris and death due to ischemic heart disease: An epidemiological study in Israeli collective settlements (kibbutzim). *Journal of Chronic Diseases*, 27, 217–33.

Bruun, K., Edwards, G., Lumio, M., Mäkelä, K., Pan, L., Popham, R.E., Room, R., Schmidt, W., Skog, O.-J., Sulkunen, P. and Österberg, E. (1975). *Alcohol control policies and public health perspective*, Vol. 25. Helsinki: Finnish Foundation for Alcohol Studies.

Byrne, D. (1961). The repression – sensitization scale: Rationale, reliability and validity. *Journal of Personality*, 29, 334–49.

Byrne, D.G., Whyte, H.M. and Butler, K.L. (1981). Illness behavior and outcome following survived myocardial infarction: A prospective study. *Journal of Psychosomatic Research*, 25, 97–107.

Caddy, G.R. (1978). Toward a multivariate analysis of alcohol abuse. In P.E. Nathan, G.A. Marlatt and T. Loberg (Eds), *Alcoholism: New directions in behavioral research*. New York: Plenum Press.

Caddy, G.R. and Block, T. (1983). Behavioral treatment methods for alcoholism. In M. Galanter (Ed.), *Recent developments in alcoholism*, Vol. 1. New York: Plenum Press.

Cannon, W.B. (1929). *Bodily changes in pain, hunger, fear, and rage*. Boston, MA: C.T. Branford.

Caplan, R.D. (1983). Person-environment fit: Past, present and future. In C.L. Cooper (Ed.), *Stress Research*, pp. 35–78. New York: Wiley.

Cappell, H. and Greeley, J. (1987). Alcohol and tension reduction: An update on research and theory. In H.T. Blane and K.E. Leonard (Eds), *Psychological theories of drinking and alcoholism*, pp. 15–54. New York: Guilford Press.

Cappell, H. and Herman, C.P. (1972). Alcohol and tension reduction: A review. *Quarterly Journal of Studies on Alcohol*, 33, 33–64.

Carmody, T.P., Brischetto, C.S., Matarazzo, J.D., O'Donnell, R.P. and Connor, W.E. (1985). Co-occurrent use of cigarette, alcohol, and coffee in healthy, community-living men and women. *Health Psychology*, 4, 323–35.

Carver, C.S., Pozo, C., Harris, S.D., Noriega, V., Scheir, M.F., Robinson, D.S., Ketcham, A.S., Moffat Jr, L. and Clark, K.C. (1993). How coping mediates the effect of optimism on distress: A study of women with early stage breast cancer. *Journal of Personality and Social Psychology*, 65, 375–90.

Castro, F.G., Newcomb, M.D., McCreary, C. and Baezconde-Garbanati, L. (1989). Cigarette smokers do more than just smoke cigarettes. *Health Psychology*, 8, 107–129.

Cataldo, M.F. and Coates, T.J. (Eds) (1986). *Health and industry: A behavioral medicine perspective*. New York: John Wiley.

Catania, J.A., Coates, T.J., Kegeles, S.M., Ekstrand, M., Guydish, J.R. and Bye, L.L. (1989). Implications of the AIDS risk-reduction model for the gay community: The importance of perceived sexual enjoyment and help-seeking behaviors. In V.M. Mays, G.W. Albee and

S.F. Schneider (Eds), *Primary prevention of AIDS*, pp. 242–61. Newbury Park, CA: Sage.

Catania, J.A., Gibson, D.R., Chitwood, D.D. and Coates, T.J. (1990). Methodological problems in AIDS behavioral research: Influences on measurement error and participation bias in studies of sexual behavior. *Psychological Bulletin*, 108, 339–62.

Catania, J.A., Coates, T.J., Stall, R., Bye, L., Kegeles, S.M., Capell, F., Henne, J., McKusick, L., Morin, S., Turner, H. and Pollack, I. (1991). Changes in condom use among homosexual men in San Francisco. *Health Psychology*, 10, 190–99.

Cautela, J.R. (1966). Treatment of compulsive behavior by covert sensitization. *Psychological Records*, 16, 33–41.

Centres for Disease Control (1987b). Human immuno-deficiency virus infection in the United States: A review of current knowledge. Morbidity and Mortality Weekly Report, 36 (Suppl. 5–6).

Centers for Disease Control (1980). *Risk factor update*. Atlanta, GA: US Department of Health and Human Services.

Cepeda-Benito, A. (1993). Meta-analytical review of the efficacy of nicotine chewing gum in smoking treatment programs. *Journal of Consulting and Clinical Psychology*, 61, 822–30.

Chaiken, S. (1980). Heuristic versus systematic information processing and the use of source versus message cues in persuasion. *Journal of Personality and Social Psychology*, 39, 725–66.

Chaisson, R.E., Moss, A.R., Onishi, R., Osmond, D. and Carlson, J.R. (1987). Human immunodeficiency virus infection in heterosexual intravenous drug users in San Francisco. *American Journal of Public Health*, 77, 169–72.

Chaney, E.F., O'Leary, M.R. and Marlatt, G.A. (1978). Skill training with alcoholics. *Journal of Consulting and Clinical Psychology*, 46, 1092–104.

Cheek, F.E., Franks, C.M., Laucious, J. and Burtle, U. (1971). Behavior modification training for wives of alcoholics. *Quarterly Journal of Studies on Alcohol*, 32, 456–61.

Christophersen, E.R. (1989). Injury contol. *American Psychologist*, 44, 237–41.

Chu, G.C. (1966). Fear arousal, efficacy and imminency, *Journal of Personality and Social Psychology*, 4, 517–23.

Clark, W.B. and Midanik, L. (1982). Alcohol use and alcohol problems among U.S. adults: Results of the 1979 national survey. In National Institute of Alcohol Abuse and Alcoholism (Ed.), *Alcohol consumption and related problems*, pp. 3–52. Alcohol and Health Monograph No. 1. Washington, DC: DHHS.

Cleary, P.D., Hitchcock, J.L., Semmer, N., Flinchbaugh, L.J. and Pinney, J.M. (1988). Adolescent smoking: Research and health policy. *The Milbank Quarterly*, 66, 137–71.

Coates, T., Stall, R., Catania, J., Dolcini, P. and Hoff, C. (1989). Prevention of HIV infection in high risk groups. In P. Volberding and M. Jacobson (Eds), *1989 AIDS clinical review*. New York: Marcel Dekker.

Cobb, S. (1976). Social support as a moderator of life stress. *Psychosomatic Medicine*, 38, 300–314.

Cobb, S. and Lindemann, E. (1943). Neuropsychiatric observations after the Coconut Grove fire. *Annals of Surgery*, 117, 814–24.

Cohen, L.H. (1988). Measurement of life events. In L.H. Cohen (Ed.), *Life events and psychological functioning*, pp. 11–30. Beverly Hills, CA: Sage.

Cohen, S. (1988). Psychological models of the role of social support in the etiology of physical disease. *Health Psychology*, 7, 269–97.

Cohen, S. and Edwards, J.R. (1989). Personality characteristics as moderators of the relationship between stress and disorder. In R.W.J. Neufeld (Ed.), *Advances in the investigation of psychological stress*, pp. 235–83. New York: John Wiley.

Cohen, S. and McKay, G. (1984). Social support, stress, and the buffering hypothesis: A theoretical analysis. In A. Baum, J.E. Singer and S.E. Taylor (Eds), *Handbook of psychology and health*, Vol. 4, pp. 253–67. Hillsdale, NJ: Laurence Erlbaum Associates Inc.

Cohen, S. and Williamson, G.M. (1988). Perceived stress in a probability sample of the United States. In S. Spacapan and S. Oskamp (Eds), *The social psychology of health*, pp. 17–67. Newbury Park, CA: Sage.

Cohen, S. and Williamson, G.M. (1991). Stress and infectious disease in humans. *Psychological Bulletin*, 109, 5–24.

Cohen, S. and Wills, T.A. (1985). Stress, social support, and the buffering hypothesis. *Psychological Bulletin*, 98, 310–357.

Cohen, S., Mermelstein, R., Kamarck, T. and Hoberman, H.N. (1985). Measuring the functional components of social support. In I.G. Sarason and B.R. Sarason (Eds), *Social support: Theory, research, and applications*, pp. 73–94. Dordrecht: Martinus Nijhoff.

Cohen, S., Lichtenstein, E., Prochaska, J.O., Rossi, J.S., Gritz, E.R., Carr, C.R., Orleans, C.R., Schoenbach, V.J., Biener, L., Abrams, D., DiClemente, C., Curry, S., Marlatt, G.A., Cummings, K.M., Emont, S.L., Giovino, G. and Ossip-Klein, D. (1989). Debunking myths about self-quitting. *American Psychologist*, 44, 1355–65.

Committee on Trauma Research (1985). *Injury in America: A continuing public health problem*. Washington, DC: National Academy Press.

Condiotte, M.M. and Lichtenstein, E. (1981). Self-efficacy and relapse in smoking cessation programs. *Journal of Consulting and Clinical Psychology*, 49, 648–58.

Cook, P.J. (1981). The effect of liquor taxes on drinking, cirrhosis, and auto accidents. In M.H. Moore and D.R. Gerstein (Eds), *Alcohol and public policy: Beyond the shadow of prohibition*, pp. 255–85. Washington, DC: National Academy Press.

Cook, P.J. (1982). Alcohol taxes as a public health measure. *British Journal of Addiction*, 77, 245–50.

Costello, R.M. (1975a). Alcoholism treatment and evaluation: In search of methods. *International Journal of Addictions*, 10, 251–75.

Costello, R.M. (1975b). Alcoholism treatment and evaluation: In search of methods. II. Collation of two-year follow-up studies. *International Journal of Addictions*, 10, 857–67.

Craighead, L.W. (1984). Sequencing of behavior therapy and pharmacotherapy for obesity. *Journal of Consulting and Clinical Psychology*, 52, 190–99.

Craighead, L.W., Stunkard, A.J. and O'Brien, R. (1981). Behavior therapy and pharmacotherapy for obesity. *Archives of General Psychiatry*, 38, 763–8.

Cummings, C., Gordon, J.F. and Marlatt, G.A. (1980). Relapse: prevention and prediction. In W.R. Miller (Ed.) *The addictive behaviors: Treatment of alcoholism, drug abuse, smoking and obesity*, pp. 291–321. New York: Pergamon.

Curran, J.W., Jaffe, H.W., Hardy, A.M., Morgan, W.M., Selik, R.M. and Dondero, P.J. (1988). Epidemiology of HIV infection and AIDS in the United States. *Science*, 239, 610–16.

Dahlkoetter, J.A., Callaghan, E.J. and Linton, J. (1979). Obesity and the unbalanced energy equation: Exercise versus eating habit change. *Journal of Consulting and Clinical Psychology*, 47, 898–905.

Dawber, T.R. (1980). *The Framingham study*. Cambridge, MA: Harvard University Press.

de Lint, J. (1976). Epidemiological aspects of alcoholism. *International Journal of Mental Health*, 5, 29–51.

DeLongis, A., Coyne, J.C., Dakof, G., Folkman, S. and Lazarus, R.S. (1982). Relationship of daily hassles, uplifts, and major life events to health status. *Health Psychology*, 1, 119–36.

Des Jarlais, D.C. and Friedman, S.R. (1988). The psychology of preventing AIDS among intravenous drug users: A social learning conceptualization. *American Psychologist*, 43, 865–70.

Des Jarlais, D.C., Friedman, S.R. and Hopkins, W. (1985). Risk reduction for the acquired immunodeficiency syndrome among intravenous drug users. *Annals of Internal Medicine*, 103, 755–9.

Detels, R., English, P., Visscher, B.R., Jacobson, L., Kingsley, L.A., Chmiel, J.S., Dudley, J.P., Eldred, L.J. and Ginzburg, H.M. (1989). Seroconversion, sexual activity and condom use among 2915 HIV seronegative men followed for up to three years. *Journal of Acquired Immune Deficiency Syndromes*, 2, 77–83.

Devor, E.J. and Cloninger, C.R. (1989). Genetics of alcoholism. *Annual Review of Genetics*, 23, 19–36.

de Wit, J.B.F., Kok, G.J., Timmermans, C.A.M. and Wijnsma, P. (1990). Determinanten van veilig vrijen en condoomgebruik bij jongeren. *Gedrag en Gezondheid*, 18, 121–33.

de Wit, J.B.F., de Vroome, E.M.M., Sandfort, T.G.M., van Griensven, G.J.P., Coutinho, R.A. and Tielman, R.A.P. (1992). Safe sexual practices not reliably maintained by homosexual men. *American Journal of Public Health*, 82, 615–16.

de Wit, J.B.F., van Griensven, G.J.P., Sandfort, T.G.M. and Coutinho, R.A. (1993a). Toename van onveilig seksueel gedrag onder homoseksuele mannen in Amsterdam. *Nederlands Tijdschrift voor Geneeskunde*, 137, 209–211.

de Wit, J.B.F., Sandfort, T.G.M., de Vroome, E., van Griensven, G.J.P. and Kok, G. (1993b). The effectiveness of the use of condoms among homosexual men. *AIDS*, 7, 751–2.

Dimsdale, J.E. and Herd, J.A. (1982). Variability of plasma lipids in response to emotional arousal. *Psychosomatic Medicine*, 44, 413–30.

Dishman, R.K. (1982). Compliance/adherence in health-related exercise. *Health Psychology*, 1, 237–67.

Dishman, R.K. and Gettman, L.R. (1980). Psychobiologic influences on exercise adherence. *Journal of Sport Psychology*, 2, 295–310.

Dishman, R.K. and Ickes, W.J. (1981). Self-motivation and adherence to therapeutic exercise. *Journal of Behavioral Medicine*, 4, 421–38.

Dishman, R.K., Ickes, W.J. and Morgan, W.P. (1980). Self-motivation and adherence to habitual physical activity. *Journal of Applied Social Psychology*, 10, 115–31.

Dohrenwend, B.P. (1973). Social status and stressful life events. *Journal of Personality and Social Psychology*, 28, 225–35.

Dohrenwend, B.P. and Shrout, P.E. (1985). "Hassles" in the conceptualization and measurement of life stress variables. *American Psychologist*, 40, 780–85.

Dohrenwend, B.S., Krasnoff, L., Askenasy, A.R. and Dohrenwend, B.P. (1978). Exemplification of a method for scoring life events: The PERI-Life-Events-Scale. *Journal of Health and Social Behavior*, 19, 205–229.

Dohrenwend, B.S., Dohrenwend, B.P., Dodson, M. and Shrout, P.E. (1984). Symptoms, hassles, social supports, and life events: Problem of confounded measures. *Journal of Abnormal Psychology*, 93, 222–30.

Doyne, E.J., Ossip-Klein, D.J., Bowman, E.D., Osborn, K.M., McDougall-Wilson, I.B. and Neimeyer, R.A. (1987). Running versus weight lifting in the treatment of depression. *Journal of Clinical and Consulting Psychology*, 55, 748–54.

Duddleston, A.K. and Bennion, M. (1970). Effect of diet and/or exercise on obese college women: Weight loss and serum lipids. *Journal of the American Dietic Association*, 56, 126–9.

Dunkel-Schetter, C. and Bennett, T.L. (1990). Differentiating the cognitive and behavioral aspects of social support. In B.R. Sarason, I.G. Sarason and G.R. Pierce (Eds), *Social support: An interactional view*, pp. 267–96. New York: John Wiley.

Duval, S. and Wicklund, R.A. (1973). *A theory of objective self-awareness*. New York: Academic Press.

Eagly, A.H. and Chaiken, S. (1993). *The psychology of attitudes*. Fort Worth, TX: Harcourt Brace Jovanovich.

Egger, G., Fitzgerald, W., Frape, G., Monaem, A., Rubinstein, P., Tyler, C. and McKay, B. (1983). Result of large scale media antismoking campaign in Australia: North Coast "Quit For Life" Programme. *British Medical Journal*, 286, 1125–8.

Ekstrand, M.L. and Coates, T.J. (1990). Maintenance of safer sexual behaviors and predictors of risky sex: The San Francisco men's health study. *American Journal of Public Health*, 80, 973–7.

Elkins, R.L. (1980). Covert sensitization treatment for alcoholism: Contributions of successful conditioning to subsequent abstinence maintenance. *Addictive Behaviors*, 5, 67–89.

Endler, N.S. and Parker, J.D.A. (1990). Multidimensional assessment of coping: A critical evaluation. *Journal of Personality and Social Psychology*, 58, 844–54.

Engel, G.L. (1977). The need for a new medical model: A challenge for biomedicine. *Science*, 196, 129–36.

Epstein, S. (1973). The self-concept revisited, or a theory of a theory. *American Psychologist*, 28, 404–416.

Epstein, S. (1979). The stability of behavior. On predicting most of the people much of the time. *Journal of Personality and Social Psychology*, 37, 1097–126.

Epstein, S. (1991). Constructive thinking and mental and physical well-being. In L. Montada, S.-H. Filipp and M.J. Lerner (Eds), *Life crises and experiences of loss in adulthood*, pp. 385–409. Hillsdale, NJ: Laurence Erlbaum Associates Inc.

Eriksen, M.P., LeMaistre, C.A. and Newell, G.R. (1988). Health hazards of passive smoking. *Annual Review of Public Health*, 9: 47–70.

Evans, R.I. (1976). Smoking in children: Developing a social psychological strategy of deterrence. *Preventive Medicine*, 5, 122–7.

Evans, R.I., Rozelle, R.M., Mittelmark, M.D., Hansen, W.B., Wane, A.L. and Havis, J. (1978). Deterring the onset of smoking in children: Knowledge of immediate physiological effects and coping with peer pressure, media pressure, and parent modelling. *Journal of Applied Social Psychology*, 8, 126–35.

Eysenck, H.J. (1965). *Smoking, health and personality*. New York: Basic Books.

Eysenck, H.J. (1980). *The courses and effects of smoking*. London: Temple Smith.

Farquhar, J.W., Maccoby, N., Wood, P.D., Alexander, J.K., Breitrose, H., Brown, B.W., Jr, Haskell, W.L., McAlister, A.L., Meyer, A.J., Nash, J.D. and Stern, M.P. (1977). Community education for cardiovascular health. *Lancet*, 1, 1192–5.

Fazio, R.H. (1986). How do attitudes guide behavior? In R.M. Sorrentino and E.T. Higgins (Eds), *Handbook of motivation and cognition: Foundations of social behavior*, pp. 204–243. New York: Guilford Press.

Fazio, R.H. (1990). Multiple processes by which attitudes guide behavior: The MODE model as an integrative framework. In M.P. Zanna (Ed.), *Advances in experimental social psychology*, Vol. 23, pp. 75–109. San Diego: Academic Press.

Fazio, R.H., and Williams, C.J. (1986). Attitude accessibility as a moderator of the attitude–perception and attitude–behavior relations: An investigation of the 1984 presidential election. *Journal of Personality and Social Psychology*, 51, 505–514.

Fazio, R.H., Chen, J., McDonel, E.C. and Sherman, S.J. (1982). Attitude accessibility, attitude–behavior consistency, and the strength of the object evaluation association. *Journal of Experimental Social Psychology*, 18, 339–57.

Ferster, C.B., Nurnberger, J.I. and Levitt, E.B. (1962). The control of eating. *Journal of Mathetics*, 1, 87–109.

Festinger, L. (1954). A theory of social comparison processes. *Human Relations*, 7, 117–40.

Fhanér, G. and Hane, M. (1979). Seat belts: Opinion effects of law-induced use. *Journal of Applied Psychology*, 64, 205–212.

Fielding, J.E. (1985a). Smoking: Health effects and control. *New England Journal of Medicine*, 313, 491–8.

Fielding, J.E. (1985b). Smoking: Health effects and control. *New England Journal of Medicine*, 313, 555–61.

Fielding, J.E. (1986). Evaluations, results and problems of worksite health promotion. In M.F. Cataldo and T.J. Coates (Eds), *Health and industry*, pp. 373–96. New York: John Wiley.

Fielding, J.E. (1991). The challenge of work-place health promotion. In S.M. Weiss, J.E. Fielding and A. Baum (Eds), *Perspectives in behavioral medicine*, pp. 13–28. Hillsdale, NJ: Lawrence Erlbaum Associates Inc.

Fielding, J.E. and Piserchia, P.V. (1989). Frequency of worksite health promotion activities. *American Journal of Public Health*, 78, 16–20.

Fineberg, H.V. (1988). Education to prevent AIDS: Prospects and obstacles. *Science*, 239, 592–6.

Fishbein, M. and Ajzen, I. (1975). *Belief, attitude, intention, and behavior: An introduction to theory and research*. Reading, MA: Addison-Wesley.

Fisher, J.D. and Fisher, W.A. (1992). Changing Aids-risk behavior. *Psychological Bulletin*, 111, 455–74.

Flay, B.R. (1985). Psychosocial approaches to smoking prevention: A review of findings. *Health Psychology*, 4, 449–88.

Fleischer, G.A. (1972). *An experiment in the use of broadcast media in highway safety.* Los Angeles: University of Southern California, Department of Industrial Systems Engineering.

Folkins, C.H. and Syme, W.E. (1981). Physical fitness training and mental health. *American Psychologist*, 36, 373–89.

Folkman, S. and Lazarus, R.S. (1980). An analysis of coping in a middle-aged community sample. *Journal of Health and Social Behavior*, 21, 219–39.

Folkman, S., Lazarus, R.S., Dunkel-Schetter, C., DeLongis, A. and Gruen, R. (1986a). The dynamics of a stressful encounter. *Journal of Personality and Social Psychology*, 50, 992–1003.

Folkman, S., Lazarus, R.S., Gruen, R.J. and DeLongis, A. (1986b). Appraisal, coping, health status and psychological symptoms. *Journal of Personality and Social Psychology*, 50, 571–9.

Ford, T.E., and Kruglanski, A.W. (in press). Effects of epistemic motivations on the use of accessible constructs in social judgement. *Personality and Social Psychology Bulletin.*

Försterling, F. (1988). *Attribution theory in clinical psychology.* Chichester: John Wiley.

Foxx, R.M. and Brown, R.A. (1979). Nicotine fading and self-monitoring for cigarette abstinence or controlled smoking. *Journal of Applied Behavior Analysis*, 12, 111–25.

French, J.R.P., Jr. and Kahn, R.L. (1962). A problematic approach to studying the industrial environment and mental health. *Journal of Social Issues*, 18, 1–47.

Friedland, G.H. and Klein, R.S. (1987). Transmission of the HIV. *New England Journal of Medicine*, 317, 1125–35.

Fries, J.F., Green, L.W. and Levine, S. (1989). Health promotion and the compression of morbidity. *Lancet*, i, 481–83.

Frost, C.D., Law, M.R. and Wald, N.J. (1991). Analysis of observational data within populations. *British Medical Journal*, 302, 815–18.

Fryer, D. (1988). The experience of unemployment in social context. In S. Fisher and J. Reason (Eds), *Handbook of life stress, cognition and health*, pp. 211–38. Chichester: John Wiley.

Funk, S.C. and Houston, B.K. (1987). A critical analysis of the hardiness scale's validity and utility. *Journal of Personality and Social Psychology*, 53, 572–8.

Furst, C.J. (1983). Estimating alcoholic prevalence. In M. Galanter (Ed.), *Recent developments in alcoholism*, Vol. 1. New York: Plenum Press.

Ganellen, R.J. and Blaney, P.H. (1984). Hardiness and social support as moderators of the effects of life stress. *Journal of Personality and Social Psychology*, 47, 156–63.

Garb, J.R., Garb, J.L. and Stunkard, A.J. (1974). Effectiveness of self-help groups in obesity. *Archives of Internal Medicine*, **134**, 716–20.

Garfinkel, L., Auerbach, O. and Joubert, L. (1985). Involuntary smoking and lung cancer: A case-control study. *Journal of the National Cancer Institute*, **75**, 463–9.

Garrow, J. (1974). *Energy balance and obesity in man*. New York: Elsevier.

George, W.H. and Marlatt, G.A. (1983). Alcoholism: The evolution of a behavioral perspective. In M. Galanter (Ed.), *Recent developments in alcoholism*, Vol. 1, pp. 105–138. New York: Plenum Press.

Glaser, R., Kiecolt-Glaser, J.K., Speicher, C.E. and Holliday, J.E. (1985). Stress, loneliness, and changes in herpesvirus latency. *Journal of Behavioral Medicine*, **8**, 249–60.

Glasgow, R.E. and Lichtenstein, E. (1987). Longterm effects of behavioral smoking cessation interventions. *Behavior Therapy*, **18**, 297–324.

Goldberg, E.L. and Comstock, G.W. (1976). Life events and subsequent illness. *American Journal of Epidemiology*, **104**, 146–58.

Goldman, L. and Cook, E.F. (1984). The decline in ischaemic heart disease mortality rates: An analysis of the comparative efforts of medical interventions and changes in lifestyle. *Annals of Internal Medicine*, **101**, 825–36.

Goldman, R., Jaffa, M. and Schachter, S. (1968). Yom Kippur, Air France, dormitory food and the eating behavior of obese and normal persons. *Journal of Personality and Social Psychology*, **10**, 117–23.

Goodwin, D.W., Schulsinger, F., Hermansen, L., Guze, S.B. and Winokur, G. (1973). Alcohol problems in adoptees raised apart from alcoholic biological parents. *Archives of General Psychiatry*, **28**, 238–43.

Goodwin, D.W., Schulsinger, F., Moller, N., Hermansen, L., Winokur, G., and Guze, S.B. (1974). Drinking problems in adopted and nonadopted sons of alcoholics. *Archives of General Psychiatry*, **31**, 164–9.

Graham, J.D. (1993). Injuries from traffic crashes: Meeting the challenge. *Annual Review of Public Health*, **14**, 515–43.

Greenwald, A.G. (1968). Cognitive learning, cognitive response to persuasion, and attitude change. In A.G. Greenwald, T.C. Brock and T.M. Ostrom (Eds), *Psychological foundations of attitudes*, pp. 147–70. San Diego, CA: Academic Press.

Greenwald, P., Sondik, E. and Lynch, B.S. (1986). Diet and chemoprevention in NCI's research strategy to achieve national cancer control objectives. *Annual Review of Public Health*, **7**, 267–92.

Grimsmo, A., Helgesen, G. and Borchgrevink, C. (1981). Short-term and long-term effects of lay groups on weight reduction. *British Medical Journal*, **283**, 1093–5.

Grunberg, N.E. (1991). Cigarette smoking at work: Data, issues, and models. In S.M. Weiss, J.E. Fielding and A. Baum (Eds), *Perspectives in behavioral medicine: Health at work*, pp. 75–98. Hillsdale, NJ: Lawrence Erlbaum Associates Inc.

Haberman, P.W. and Baden, M.M. (1978). *Alcohol, other drugs and violent death*. New York: Oxford University Press.

Haddon, W., Jr and Baker, S.P. (1981). Injury control. In D. Clark and B. McMahon (Eds), *Preventive and community medicine*, pp. 109–140. Boston, MA: Little, Brown.

Haddon, W., Jr, Valien, P., McCarroll, J.R. and Umberger, C.J. (1961). A controlled investigation of the characteristics of adult pedestrians fatally injured by motor vehicles in Manhattan. *Journal of Chronic Diseases*, 14, 655–678.

Haddy, F.J. (1991). Roles of sodium, potassium, calcium, and natriuretic factors in hypertension. *Hypertension*, 18: 179–83 (suppl. III).

Hahn, M.E. (1966). *California-Life-Goals-Evaluation-Schedule*. Palo Alto, CA: Western Psychological Services.

Hall, S.M., Hall, R.G. and Ginsberg, D. (1990). Cigarette dependence. In A.S. Bellack, M. Hersen and A.E. Kazdin (Eds), *International handbook of behavior modification and therapy*, 2nd edn, pp. 437–47. New York: Plenum Press.

Harackiewicz, J.M., Sansone, C., Blair, L.W., Epstein, J.A. and Manderlink, G. (1987). Attributional processes in behavior change and maintenance: Smoking cessation and continued abstinence. *Journal of Consulting and Clinical Psychology*, 55, 372–8.

Harris, J.E. (1982). Increasing the federal excise tax on cigarettes. *Journal of Health Economics*, 1, 117–20.

Harris, M.B. and Hallbauer, E.S. (1973). Self-directed weight control through eating and exercise. *Behavior Research and Therapy*, 11, 523–9.

Heather, N. and Robertson, I. (1983). *Controlled drinking*. London: Methuen.

Heatherton, T.F., Herman, C.P. and Polivy, J. (1991). Effects of physical threat and ego threat on eating behavior. *Journal of Personality and Social Psychology*, 60, 138–43.

Heider, F. (1958). *The psychology of interpersonal relations*. New York: John Wiley.

Helsing, K.J., Sandler, D.P., Comstock, G.W. and Chee, E. (1988). Heart disease mortality in non-smokers living with smokers. *American Journal of Epidemiology*, 127, 915–22.

Hennekens, C.H., Willet, W., Rosner, B., Cole, D.S. and Mayrent, S.L. (1979). Effects of beer, wine, and liquor in coronary deaths. *Journal of the American Medical Association*, 242, 1973–4.

Herd, A.J. (1978). Physiological correlates of coronary-prone behavior. In T.M. Dembrowski, S.M. Weiss, J.L. Shields, S.G. Haynes and M. Feinleib (Eds), *Coronary-prone behavior*. New York: Springer.

Herman, C.P. and Mack, D. (1975). Restrained and unrestrained eating. *Journal of Personality*, 43, 647–60.

Herman, C.P. and Polivy, J. (1975). Anxiety, restraint and eating behavior. *Journal of Abnormal Psychology*, 84, 666–72.

Herman, C.P. and Polivy, J. (1984). A boundary model for the regulation of eating. In A.J. Stunkard and E. Stellar (Eds), *Eating and its disorders*, pp. 141–56. New York: Raven Press.

Herman, C.P., Polivy, J., Lank, C.L. and Heatherton, T.F. (1987). Anxiety, hunger, and eating. *Journal of Abnormal Psychology*, 96, 264–9.

Hibscher, J.A. and Herman, C.P. (1977). Obesity, dieting, and the expression of "obese" characteristics. *Journal of Comparative and Physiological Psychology*, 91, 374–80.

Higgins, R.L. and Marlatt, G.A. (1975). Fear of interpersonal evaluation as a determinant of alcohol consumption in male social drinkers. *Journal of Abnormal Psychology*, 84, 644–51.

Hill, S., Steinhauer, S.R. and Zubin, J. (1986). Biological markers for alcoholism: A vulnerability model conceptualization. In R.A. Dienstbier (Ed.), *Nebraska symposium on motivation*, pp. 207–256. Lincoln: Nebraska University Press.

Hiroto, D.S. (1974). Locus of control and learnt helplessness. *Journal of Experimental Psychology*, 102, 187–93.

Hiroto, D.S. and Seligman, M.E.P. (1975). Generality of learnt helplessness in man. *Journal of Personality and Social Psychology*, 32, 311–27.

Hirsch, J. and Knittle, J.L. (1970). Cellularity of obese and nonobese human adipose tissue. *Federation Proceedings*, 29, 1516–21.

Hirschman, R.S. and Leventhal, H. (1989). Preventing smoking behavior in schoolchildren: An initial test of a cognitive-development program. *Journal of Applied Social Psychology*, 19, 559–583.

Holme, I. (1990). An analysis of randomized trials evaluating the effect of cholesterol reduction on total mortality and coronary heart disease incidence. *Circulation*, 82, 1916–24.

Holmes, T.H. and Masuda, M. (1974). Life change and illness susceptibility. In W.S. Dohrenwend and B.P. Dohrenwend (Eds), *Stress for life events*, pp. 45–72. New York: John Wiley.

Holmes, T.H. and Rahe, R.H. (1967). The social readjustment rating-scale. *Journal of Psychosomatic Research*, 11, 213–18.

House, J.S. (1981). *Workstress and social support*. Reading, MA: Addison-Wesley.

House, J.S. and Kahn, R.L. (1985). Measures and concepts of social support. In S. Cohen and S.L. Syme (Eds), *Social support and health*, pp. 83–108. Orlando, FL: Academic Press.

House, J.S., Robbins, C. and Metzner, H.L. (1982). The association of social relationships and activities with mortality: Prospective evidence from the Tecumseh Community Health Study. *American Journal of Epidemiology*, 116, 123–40.

House, J.S., Landis, K.R. and Umberson, D. (1988). Social relationships and health. *Science*, 241, 540–45.

Houston, D.A. and Fazio, R.H. (1989). Biased processing as a function of attitude accessibility: Making objective judgements subjectively. *Social Cognition*, 7, 51–66.

Hull, J.G. (1981). A self-awareness model of the causes and effects of alcohol consumption. *Journal of Abnormal Psychology*, 90, 586–600.

Hull, J.G. (1987). Self-awareness model. In H.T. Blane and K.E. Leonard (Eds), *Psychological theories of drinking and alcoholism*, pp. 272–304. New York: Guilford Press.

Hull, J.G. and Bond, C.F., Jr (1986). Social behavioral consequences of alcohol consumption and expectancy: A meta-analysis. *Psychological Bulletin*, 99, 347–60.

Hull, J., Levenson, R., Young, R. and Sher, K. (1983). The self-awareness-reducing effects of alcohol consumption. *Journal of Personality and Social Psychology*, 44, 461–73.

Hull, J., van Teuren, R. and Virnelli, S. (1987). Hardiness and health: A critique and alternative approach. *Journal of Personality and Social Psychology*, 53, 518–30.

Hulley, S.B. and Hearst, N. (1989). The worldwide epidemiology and prevention of AIDS. In V.M. Mays, G.W. Albee and S.F. Schneider (Eds), *Primary prevention of AIDS*, pp. 47–71. Newbury Park, CA: Sage.

Humble, C.G., Samet, J.M. and Pathak, D.R. (1987). Marriage to a smoker and lung cancer risk. *American Journal of Public Health*, 77, 598–602.

Hunt, G.M. and Azrin, N.H. (1973). A community-reinforcement approach to alcoholism. *Behaviour, Research and Therapy*, 11, 91–104.

Hurley, J. and Horowitz, J. (Eds) (1990). *Alcohol and health*. New York: Hemisphere.

Ikard, F. and Tomkins, S. (1973). The experience of affect as a determinant of smoking behavior: A series of validity studies. *Journal of Abnormal Psychology*, 81, 172–81.

Ikard, F.F., Green, D.E. and Horn, D.A. (1969). A scale to differentiate between types of smoking as related to management of affect. *International Journal of the Addictions*, 4, 649–59.

Imber, S., Schultz, E., Funderburk, F., Allen, R. and Flamer, R. (1976). The fate of the untreated alcoholic. *Journal of Nervous and Mental Disease*, 162, 238–47.

Ingram, R.E. and Scott, W.D. (1990). Cognitive behavior therapy. In A.S. Bellack, M. Hersen and A.E. Kazdin (Eds), *International handbook of behavior modification and therapy*, 2nd edn, pp. 53–65. New York: Plenum Press.

Istvan, J. and Matarazzo, J.D. (1984). Tobacco, alcohol, and caffeine use: A review of their interrelationships. *Psychological Bulletin*, 95, 301–326.

Jackson, R., Scragg, R. and Beaglehole, R. (1991). Alcohol consumption and risk of coronary heart disease. *British Medical Journal*, 303, 211–16.

Jacobs, D.R., Jr (1993). Why is low blood cholesterol associated with risk of nonatherosclerotic disease death? *Annual Review of Public Health*, 14, 95–114.

Janz, N.K. and Becker, M.H. (1984). The health belief model: A decade later. *Health Education Quarterly*, 11, 1–47.

Jeffery, R.W. (1989). Risk behaviors and health: Contrasting individual and population perspectives. *American Psychology*, 44, 1194–1202.

Jeffery, R.W., Wing, R.R. and Stunkard, A.J. (1978). Behavioral treatment of obesity: The state of the art in 1976. *Behavior Therapy*, 9, 189–99.

Jellinek, E.M. (1960). *The disease concept of alcoholism*. Highland Park, NJ: Hillhouse.

Jepson, C. and Chaiken, S. (1990). Chronic issue-specific fear inhibits systematic processing of persuasive communications. *Journal of Social Behavior and Personality*, 5, 61–84.

Johnson, J.A. and Oksanen, E.H. (1977). Estimations of demand for alcoholic beverages in Canada from pooled time series and cross sections. *Review of Economics and Statistics*, 59, 113–18.

Jonas, K. (1993). Expectancy-value models of health behaviour: An analysis by conjoint measurement. *European Journal of Social Psychology*, 23, 167–85.

Jonas, K., Stroebe, W. and Eagly, A. (1993). Adherence to an exercise program. Unpublished manuscript, University of Tübingen.

Jose, W.S., II and Anderson, D.R. (1991). Control data's Staywell Program: A health cost management strategy. In S.M. Weiss, J.E. Fielding and A. Baum (Eds), *Perspectives in behavioral medicine: Health at work*, pp. 75–98. Hillsdale, NJ: Lawrence Erlbaum Associates Inc.

Kannel, W.B., Castelli, W.P., Gordon, T. and McNamara, P.M. (1971). Serum cholesterol lipoproteins and risk of heart diseases: The Framingham Study. *Annals of Internal Medicine*, 24, 1–12.

Kanner, A.D., Coyne, J.C., Schaever, C. and Lazarus, R.S. (1981). Comparison of two modes of stress measurement: Daily hassles and uplifts versus major life events. *Journal of Behavioral Medicine*, 4, 1–39.

Kaplan, R.M. (1984). The connection between clinical health promotion and health status: A critical review. *American Psychologist*, 39, 755–65.

Kaplan, R.M. (1985). Behavioural epidemiology, health promotion and health services. *Medical Care*, 23, 562–83.

Kaplan, R.M. (1986). Dietary aspects in the treatment of hypertension. *Annual Review of Public Health*, 7, 503–520.

Kaplan, R.M. (1988). The value dimension in studies of health promotion. In S. Spacapan and S. Oskamp (Eds), *The social psychology of health*. Beverly Hills, CA: Sage.

Kasl, S.V., Evans, A.A. and Niederman, J.C. (1979). Psychological risk factors in the development of infectious mononucleosis. *Psychosomatic Medicine*, 41, 445–66.

Keesey, R.E. (1980). The regulation of body weight: A set-point analysis. In A.J. Stunkard (Ed.), *Obesity*, pp. 144–65. Philadelphia, PA: W.B. Saunders.

Keesey, R.E. (1986). A set-point theory of obesity. In K.D. Brownell and J.P. Foreyt (Eds), *The physiology, psychology, and treatment of eating disorders*, pp. 63–87. New York: Basic Books.

Kelly, J.A., St. Lawrence, J.S., Brasfield, T.L. and Hood, H.V. (1989). Behavioral intervention to reduce AIDS risk activities. *Journal of Consulting and Clinical Psychology*, 57, 60–67.

Kendell, R.E. and Staton, M.C. (1966). The fate of untreated alcoholics. *Quarterly Journal of Studies in Alcohol*, 27, 30–41.

Kendell, R.E., de Roumanie, M. and Ritson, E.B. (1983a). The influence of an increase in exercise duty on alcohol consumption and its adverse effects. *British Medical Journal*, 287, 809–811.

Kendell, R.E., de Roumanie, M. and Ritson, E.B. (1983b). Effects of economic changes on Scottish drinking habits 1978–1982. *British Journal of Addiction*, 78, 365–79.

Kenney, W.L. (1985). Parasympathetic control of resting heart rate: Relationship to aerobic power. *Medicine and Science in Sports and Exercise*, 17, 451–5.

Kent, K.M., Smith, E.R., Redwood, D.R. and Epstein, S.E. (1973). Electrical stability of acutely ischemic myocardium: Influences of heart rate and vagal stimulation. *Circulation*, 47, 291–8.

Kent, T.H. and Hart, M.N. (1987). *Introduction to human disease*, 2nd edn. East Norwalk, CT: Appleton-Century-Crofts.

Keys, A. (1980). *Seven countries: A multivariate analysis of death and coronary heart disease*. Cambridge, MA: Harvard University Press.

Keys, A., Brozek, J., Henschel, A., Nickelson, O. and Taylor, H.L. (1950). *The biology of human starvation*, Vols 1 and 2. Minneapolis, MI: University of Minnesota Press.

Kiecolt-Glaser, J.K. and Glaser, R. (1991). Stress and immune function in humans. In R. Ader, D.L. Felten and N. Cohen (Eds), *Psychoneuroimmunology*, 2nd edn, pp. 849–67. San Diego: Academic Press.

Kiecolt-Glaser, J.K., Garner, W., Speicher, C.E., Penn, G. and Glaser, R. (1984). Psychosocial modifiers of immunocompetence in medical students. *Psychosomatic Medicine*, 46, 7–14.

Kiecolt-Glaser, J.K., Glaser, R., Shuttleworth, E.C., Dyer, C.S., Ogrocki, P. and Speicher, C.E. (1987). Chronic stress and immunity in family caregivers of Alzheimers' disease victims. *Psychosomatic Medicine*, 49, 523–35.

Kiecolt-Glaser, J.K., Kennedy, S., Malkoff, S., Fisher, L., Speicher, C.E. and Glaser, R. (1988). Marital discord and immunity in males. *Psychosomatic Medicine*, 50, 213–29.

King, A.C., Taylor, C.B., Haskell, W.L. and DeBusk, R.F. (1989). Influence of regular aerobic exercise on psychological health: A randomized, controlled trial of healthy middle-aged adults. *Health Psychology*, 8, 305–324.

Kittel, F., Kornitzer, M., Dramaix, M. and Beriot, I. (1993). Health behavior in Belgian studies: Who is doing best? Paper presented at the *European Congress of Psychology*, September 1–3, Brussels.

Klesges, R.C. and Glasgow, R.E. (1986). Smoking modification in the worksite. In M.F. Cataldo and T.J. Coates (Eds), *Health and industry: A behavioral medicine perspective*, pp. 231–54. New York: John Wiley.

Klesges, R.C., Vasey, M.M. and Glasgow, R.E. (1986). A worksite smoking modification competition: Potential for public health impact. *American Journal of Public Health*, 76, 198–200.

Klesges, R.C., Glasgow, R.E., Klesges, L.M., Morray, K. and Quale, R. (1987). Competition and relapse prevention training in worksite smoking modification. *Health Education Research: Theory and Practice*, 2, 5–14.

Knight, L. and Boland, F. (1989). Restrained eating: An experimental disentanglement of the disinhibiting variables of calories and blood type. *Journal of Abnormal Psychology*, 98, 412–20.

Kobasa, S.C. (1979). Stressful life events, personality, and health: An inquiry into hardiness. *Journal of Personality and Social Psychology*, 37, 1–11.

Kobasa, S.C. and Puccetti, M.C. (1983). Personality and social resources in stress resistance. *Journal of Personality and Social Psychology*, 45, 839–50.

Kobasa, S.C., Maddi, S.R. and Courington, S. (1981). Personality and constitution as mediators in the stress–illness relationship. *Journal of Health and Social Behavior*, 22, 368–78.

Kobasa, S.C., Maddi, S.R. and Kahn, S. (1982a). Hardiness and health: A prospective study. *Journal of Personality and Social Psychology*, 42, 168–77.

Kobasa, S.C., Maddi, S.R. and Puccetti, M.C. (1982b). Personality and exercise as buffers in the stress–illness relationship. *Journal of Behavioral Medicine*, 5, 391–404.

Kramsch, D.M., Aspen, A.J., Abramowitz, B.M., Kreimendahl, T. and Hood, W.B., Jr (1981). Reduction of coronary atherosclerosis by moderate conditioning exercise in monkeys on an atherogenic diet. *New England Journal of Medicine*, 303, 1483–9.

Krotkiewski, M., Björntorp, P., Sjöström, L. and Smith, O. (1983). Impact of obesity on metabolism in men and women: Importance of regional adipose tissue distribution. *Journal of Clinical Investigation*, 72, 1150–62.

Krüger, H. and Schmidt, F. (1989). Leichtrauchen ist kein Ausweg. *Die Medizinische Welt*, 40, 1091–4.

Kruglanski, A.W. (1989). *Lay epistemics and human knowledge: Cognitive and motivational bases*. New York: Plenum Press.

Lakey, B. and Heller, K. (1985). Response biases and the relation between negative life events and psychological symptoms. *Journal of Personality and Social Psychology*, 49, 1662–8.

Lando, H.A. (1977). Successful treatment of smokers with a broad-spectrum behavioral approach. *Journal of Consulting and Clinical Psychology*, 45, 361–6.

Larsson, B., Björntorp, P. and Tibblin, G. (1981). The health consequences of moderate obesity. *International Journal of Obesity*, 5, 97–116.

Laudenslager, M.L., Boccia, M.L. and Reite, M.L. (1993). In M. Stroebe, W. Stroebe and R. Hansson (Eds), *Handbook of bereavement: Theory, research and intervention*, 129–42. New York: Cambridge University Press.

Law, M.R., Frost, C.D. and Wald, N.J. (1991a). By how much does dietary salt reduction lower blood pressure? I: Analysis of observational data among populations. *British Medical Journal*, 302, 811–15.

Law, M.R., Frost, C.D. and Wald, N.J. (1991b). By how much does dietary salt reduction lower blood pressure? III: Analysis of data from trials of salt reduction. *British Medical Journal*, 302, 818–24.

Lazarus, A.A. (1965). Towards the understanding and effective treatment of alcoholism. *South African Medical Journal*, 39, 736–41.

Lazarus, R.S. and Folkman, S. (1984). *Stress, appraisal, and coping*. New York: Springer.

Lazarus, R.S., DeLongis, A., Folkman, S. and Gruen, R. (1985). Stress and adaptational outcomes: The problem of confounded measures. *American Psychologist*, 40, 770–79.

Ledermann, S. (1956). *Alcool, alcoolisme, alcoolisation: Donées scientifiques de caractère physiologique, économique et social*. Institut National D'Études Démographiques. Travaux et Documents, Cahier No. 29. Paris: Presses Universitaires de France.

Ledermann, S. (1964). *Alcool, alcoolisme, alcoolisation: Mortalité, morbidité, accidents du travail*. Institut National D'Études Démographiques. Travaux et Documents. Cahier No. 41. Paris: Presses Universitaires de France.

Lefebvre, R.C. (1986). Diet, lipids, and coronary heart disease. *American Psychologist*, 41, 96–8.

Lemers, F. and Voegtlin, W.L. (1950). An evaluation of the aversion treatment of alcoholism. *Quarterly Journal of Studies on Alcohol*, 11, 199–204.

Lepper, M.R. and Greene, D. (1978). *The hidden cost of reward*. New York: John Wiley.

Leventhal, H. and Avis, N. (1976). Pleasure, addiction, and habit: Factors in verbal report or factors in smoking behavior? *Journal of Abnormal Psychology*, 85, 478–88.

Leventhal, H. and Cleary, P.D. (1980). The smoking problem: A review of the research and theory in behavioral risk modification. *Psychological Bulletin*, 88, 370–405.

Leventhal, H., Fleming, R. and Glynn, K. (1988). A cognitive-developmental approach to smoking intervention. In S. Maes, C. Spielberger, P.B. Devares and I.G. Sarason (Eds), *Topics in health psychology*, pp. 79–105. New York: John Wiley.

Lew, E.A. and Garfinkel, L. (1979). Variation in mortality by weight among 750,000 men and women. *Journal of Chronic Diseases*, 32, 563–76.

Lewit, E.M. and Coate, D. (1982). The potential for using excise taxes to reduce smoking. *Journal of Health Economics*, 1, 121–45.

Lichtenstein, E. (1982). The smoking problem: A behavioral perspective. *Journal of Consulting and Clinical Psychology*, 50, 804–19.

Lichtenstien, E. and Danaher, B.G. (1975). Modification of smoking behavior: A critical analysis of theory, research, and practice. In M. Hersen, R. Eisler and P. Miller (Eds), *Progress in Behavior Modification*, Vol. 3, pp. 79–132. New York: Academic Press.

Lipid Research Clinics Program (1984a). The lipid research clinic's coronary primary prevention trial results: I. Reduction in the incidence of coronary heart disease. *Journal of the American Medical Association*, 253, 351–64.

Lipid Research Clinics Program (1984b). The lipid research clinic's coronary primary prevention trial results: II. The relationship of reduction in incidence of coronary heart disease to cholesterol lowering. *Journal of the American Medical Association*, 251, 365–74.

Liska, A.E. (1984). A critical examination of the causal structure of the Fishbein/Ajzen attitude–behavior model. *Social Psychology Quarterly*, 47, 61–74.

Litman, G.K. and Topham, A. (1980). Outcome studies on techniques in alcoholism treatment. In M. Galanter (Ed.), *Recent developments in alcoholism*, Vol. I, pp. 107–194. New York: Plenum Press.

Lloyd, R.W., Jr and Salzberg, H.C. (1975). Controlled social drinking: An alternative to abstinence as a treatment goal for some alcohol abusers. *Psychological Bulletin*, 82, 815–42.

Locke, E.A. and Latham, G.P. (1990). *A theory of goal setting and task performance*. Englewood Cliffs, NJ: Prentice-Hall.

Logue, A.W. (1986). *The psychology of eating and drinking.* New York: Freeman.

Lynch, J.J. (1970). *The broken heart: The medical consequences of loneliness.* New York: Basic Books.

Maddi, S.R., Bartone, P.T. and Puccetti, M.C. (1987). Stressful events are indeed a factor in physical illness: A reply to Schroeder and Costa (1984). *Journal of Personality and Social Psychology,* 52, 833–43.

Maddi, S.R., Kobasa, S.C. and Hoover, M. (1979). An alienation test. *Journal of Humanistic Psychology,* 19, 73–6.

Maddox, G.L., Back, K.W. and Liederman, V.R. (1968). Overweight and social deviance and disability. *Journal of Health and Social Behavior,* 9, 287–98.

Mahoney, M.J. and Mahoney, K. (1976). *Permanent weight control: A total solution to a dieter's dilemma.* New York: W.W. Norton.

Maisto, S.A., Lauerman, R. and Adesso, V.J. (1977). A comparison of two experimental studies of the role of cognitive factors in alcoholics' drinking. *Journal of Studies on Alcohol,* 38, 145–9.

Malin, H., Coakley, J., Kaelber, C., Munch, N. and Holland, W. (1982). An epidemiologic perspective on alcohol use and abuse in the United States. In National Institute of Alcohol Abuse and Alcoholism (Ed.), *Alcohol consumption and related problems,* pp. 99–153. Washington, DC: DHHS.

Manstead, A.S.R., Proffitt, C. and Smart, J.L. (1983). Predicting and understanding mother's infant-feeding intentions and behavior: Testing the theory of reasoned action. *Journal of Personality and Social Psychology,* 44, 657–71.

Marlatt, G.A. (1976). Alcohol, stress, and cognitive control. In I.S. Sarason and C.D. Spielberger (Eds), *Stress and anxiety,* Vol. 3, pp. 271–96. Washington, DC: Hemisphere.

Marlatt, G.A. (1985). Relapse prevention: Theoretical rationale and overview of the model. In G.A. Marlatt and J.R. Gordon (Eds), *Relapse prevention,* pp. 3–70. New York: Guilford Press.

Marlatt, G.A. and Gordon, J.R. (1980). Determinants of relapse: Implications for the maintenance of behavior change. In P.O. Davidson and S.M. Davidson (Eds), *Behavioral Medicine,* pp. 410–52. New York: Brunner/Mazel.

Marlatt, G.A. and Rohsenow, D.J. (1980). Cognitive processes in alcohol use: Expectancy and the balanced placebo design. In N.K. Mellow (Ed.), *Advances in substance Abuse,* Vol. 1, pp. 159–99. Greenwich, Conn: JAI Press.

Marlatt, G.A., Demming, B. and Reid, J.B. (1973). Loss of control drinking in alcoholics: An experimental analogue. *Journal of Abnormal and Social Psychology,* 81, 233–41.

Marlatt, G.A., Curry, S. and Gordon, J.R. (1988). A longitudinal analysis of unaided smoking cessation. *Journal of Consulting and Clinical Psychology*, **56**, 715–20.

Martin, J.L. (1987). The impact of AIDS on gay male sexual behavior patterns in New York City. *American Journal of Public Health*, **77**, 578–81.

Mason, J.W. (1975). A historical view of the stress field (parts I, II). *Journal of Human Stress*, **1**, 6–12, 22–36.

Matarazzo, J.D. (1984). Behavioral health: A 1990 challenge for the health sciences professions. In J.D. Matarazzo, N.E. Miller, S.M. Weiss, J.A. Herd and S.M. Weiss (Eds), *Behavioral health: A handbook of health enhancement and disease prevention*, pp. 3–40. New York: John Wiley.

McCann, I.L. and Holmes, D.S. (1984). Influence of aerobics on depression. *Journal of Personality and Social Psychology*, **46**, 1142–7.

McCarroll, J.R. and Haddon, W., Jr (1962). A controlled study of fatal motor vehicle crashes in New York City. *Journal of Chronic Diseases*, **15**, 811–22.

McClelland, D.C., Davis, W.N., Kalin, R. and Wanner, E. (1972). *The drinking man*. New York: Free Press.

McCrae, R.R. and Costa Jr, P.T. (1986). Personality, coping and coping effectiveness in an adult sample. *Journal of Personality*, **54**, 385–405.

McDonald, D.G. and Hodgdon, J.A. (1991). *Psychological effects of aerobic fitness training: Research and theory*. New York: Springer.

McGinnis, J.M., Shopland, D. and Brown, C. (1987). Tobacco and health: Trends in smoking and smokeless tobacco consumption in the United States. *Annual Review of Public Health*, **8**, 441–67.

McGuire, R.J. and Vallance, M. (1964). Aversion therapy by electric shock: A simple technique. *British Medical Journal*, **1**, 151–3.

McGuire, W.J. (1985). Attitudes and attitude change. In G. Lindzey and E. Aronson (Eds), *Handbook of social psychology*, 3rd edn, Vol. 2, pp. 233–346. New York: Random House.

McKeown, T. (1979). *The role of medicine*. Oxford: Blackwell.

McKinlay, J.B. and McKinlay, S.M. (1981). Medical measures and the decline of mortality. In P. Conrad and R. Kern (Eds), *The sociology of health and illness*, pp. 12–30. New York: St. Martins Press.

McKinnon, W., Weisse, C.S., Reynolds, C.P., Bowles, C.A. and Baum, A. (1989). Chronic stress, leukocyte subpopulations, and humoral response to latent viruses. *Health Psychology*, **8**, 389–402.

McKusick, L., Wiley, J.A., Coates, T.J., Stall, R., Saika, G., Morin, S., Charles, K., Horstman, W. and Conant, M.A. (1985a). Reported changes in the sexual behavior of men at risk for AIDS, San Francisco, 1982–84: The AIDS Behavioral Research Project. *Public Health Reports*, **100**, 622–9.

McKusick, L., Horstman, W. and Coates, T.J. (1985b). AIDS and sexual behavior reported by gay men in San Francisco. *American Journal of Public Health*, 75, 493–6.

Mechanic, D. (1978). *Medical sociology*, 2nd edn. New York: Free Press.

Mechanic, D. (1979). The stability of health and illness behavior: Results from a 16-year follow-up. *American Journal of Public Health*, 69, 1142–5.

Meichenbaum, P. (1977). *Cognitive behavior modification*. New York: Plenum Press.

Meyer, A.J., Nash, J.D., McAlister, A.L., Maccoby, N. and Farquhar, J.W. (1980). Skills training in a cardiovascular health education campaign. *Journal of Consulting and Clinical Psychology*, 48, 129–42.

Miller, P.M. (1972). The use of behavioral contracting in the treatment of alcoholism. *Behavior Therapy*, 3, 593–6.

Miller, P.M., Hersen, M., Eisler, R.M. and Hilsman, G. (1974). Effects of social stress on operant drinking of alcoholics and social drinkers. *Behavior Research and Therapy*, 12, 67–72.

Miller, S.M. (1980). Why having control reduces stress: If I can stop the roller coaster, I don't want to get off. In J. Garber and M.E.P. Seligman (Eds), *Human helplessness: Theory and applications*, pp. 71–95. New York: Academic Press.

Miller, W.R. and Hester, R.K. (1986). The effectiveness of alcoholism treatment: What research reveals. In W.R. Miller and N. Heather (Eds), *Treating addictive behaviors: Processes of change*, pp. 121–74. New York: Plenum Press.

Miller, W.R. and Munoz, R.F. (1976). *How to control your drinking?* Englewood Cliffs, NJ: Prentice-Hall.

Miller, W.R., Taylor, C.A. and West, J.C. (1980). Focused versus broad-spectrum behavior therapy for problem drinkers. *Journal of Consulting and Clinical Psychology*, 48, 590–601.

Monroe, S.M. (1983). Major and minor life events as predictors of psychological distress: Further issues and findings. *Journal of Behavioral Medicine*, 6, 189–205.

Mooney, A.J. (1982). Alcohol use. In Taylor, R.B. (Ed.), *Health promotion principles and clinical applications*, pp. 233–58. New York: Appleton.

Mooney, A.J., III and Cross, G.M. (1988). Alcoholism and substance abuse. In L.B. Taylor (Ed.), *Family medicine*, 3rd edn, pp. 690–702. New York: Springer.

Moore, M.H. and Gerstein, D.R. (Eds) (1981). *Alcohol and public policy: Beyond the shadow of prohibition*. Washington, DC: National Academy Press.

Morgan, W.P. and O'Connor, P.J. (1988). Exercise and mental health. In R.K. Dishman (Ed.), *Exercise adherence: Its impact on public health*, pp. 91–121. Champaign, IL: Human Kinetics.

Morris, J.N., Heady, J.A., Raffle, P., Roberts, C.G. and Parks, J.W. (1953).

Coronary heart disease and physical activity of work. *Lancet*, 2, 1053–7, 1111–20.

Morris, J.N., Everitt, M.G., Pollard, R. and Chave, S.P.W. (1980a). Exercise and the heart (Letter). *Lancet*, 1, 267.

Morris, J.N., Pollard, R., Everitt, M.G. and Chave, S.P.W. (1980b). Vigorous exercise in leisure-time protection against coronary heart disease. *Lancet*, 2, 1207–1210.

National Center for Health Statistics (1989). *Health, United States, 1988*. DHHS Publication No. (PHS) 89–1252. Washington, DC: US Government Printing Office.

National Safety Council (1986). *Accident facts – 1986*. Chicago, IL: National Safety Council.

Neil, W.A. and Oxendine, J.M. (1979). Exercise can promote coronary collateral development without improving perfusion of ischemic myocardium. *Circulation*, 60, 1513–19.

Nisbett, R.E. (1968). Taste, deprivation, and weight determinants of eating behavior. *Journal of Personality and Social Psychology*, 10, 107–116.

Nisbett, R.E. (1972). Hunger, obesity, and the ventromedial hypothalamus. *Psychological Review*, 79, 433–53.

Novotny, T.E., Romano, R.A., Davis, R.M. and Mills, S.L. (1992). The public health practice of tobacco control: Lessons learned and directions for the States in the 1990s. *Annual Review of Public Health*, 13, 287–318.

Oldridge, N.B. (1984). Adherence to adult exercise fitness programs. In J.D. Matarazzo, S.M. Weiss, J.A. Herd, N.E. Miller and S.M. Weiss (Eds), *Behavioral health: A handbook of health enhancement and disease prevention*, pp. 467–87. New York: John Wiley.

O'Leary, A.O. (1990). Stress, emotion, and human immune function. *Psychological Bulletin*, 108, 363–82.

Olson, J.M. and Zanna, M.P. (1982). *Predicting adherence to a program of physical exercise: An emperical study*. Toronto: Government of Ontario, Ministry of Tourism and Recreation.

Orford, J. (1985). *Excessive appetites: A psychological view of addictions*. Chichester: John Wiley.

Osborn, J.E. (1989). A risk assessment of the AIDS epidemic. In V.M. Mays, G.W. Albee and S.F. Schneider (Eds), *Primary prevention of AIDS*, pp. 23–38. Newbury Park, CA: Sage.

Osterweis, M., Solomon, T. and Green, M. (1984). *Bereavement: Reactions, consequences, and care*. Washington, DC: National Academy Press.

Paffenbarger, R.S., Jr and Hale, W.E. (1975). Work activity and coronary heart mortality. *New England Journal of Medicine*, 292, 545–50.

Paffenbarger, R.S., Jr, Wing, A.L. and Hyde, R.T. (1978). Chronic disease in former college students. XVI: Physical activity as an index of heart attack risk in college alumni. *American Journal of Epidemiology*, 108, 161–75.

Paffenbarger, R.S., Jr, Wing, A.L., Hyde, R.T. and Jung, D.L. (1983). Physical activity and incidence of hypertension in college alumni. *American Journal of Epidemiology*, 117, 245–57.

Paffenbarger, R.S., Jr, Hyde, R.T., Wing, A.L. and Hsieh, C. (1986). Cigarette smoking and cardiovascular disease. In D.G. Zaridze and R. Peto (Eds), *A major international hazard*. IARC Scientific Publication No. 74. Lyon: International Agency for Research on Cancer.

Paffenbarger, R.S., Jr and Hyde, T.T. (1988). Exercise adherence, coronary disease, and longevity. In R.K. Dishman (Ed.), *Exercise adherence: Its impact on public health*, pp. 41–73. Champaign, IL: Human Kinetics.

Parker, J.D.A. and Endler, N.S. (1992). Coping with coping assessment: A critical review. *European Journal of Personality*, 6, 321–44.

Parkes, C.M. (1986). *Bereavement: Studies of grief in adult life*. Harmondsworth: Penguin.

Parkes, C.M., Benjamin, B. and Fitzgerald, R.G. (1969). Broken heart: A statistical study of increased mortality among widowers. *British Medical Journal*, 1, 740–43.

Patrick, K., Grace, T.W. and Lovato, C.Y. (1992). Health issues for college students. *Annual Review of Public Health*, 13, 253–68.

Pennebaker, J.W. and Beall, S. (1986). Cognitive, emotional and physiological components of confiding: Behavioral inhibition and disease. (Unpublished).

Pennebaker, J.W., Kiecolt-Glaser, J. and Glaser, R. (1988). Disclosure of traumas and immune function: Health implications for psychotherapy. *Journal of Consulting and Clinical Psychology*, 56, 239–45.

Pennebaker, J.W., Colder, M. and Sharp, L.K. (1990). Accelerating the coping process. *Journal of Personality and Social Psychology*, 58, 528–37.

Pershagen, G., Hrubec, Z. and Svensson, C. (1987). Passive smoking and lung cancer in Swedish women. *American Journal of Epidemiology*, 125, 17–24.

Peterson, C. and Seligman, M.E.P. (1987). Coarse explanations as a risk factor for depression: Theory and evidence. *Psychological Review*, 91, 347–74.

Peterson, C., Seligman, M.E.P. and Vaillant, G.E. (1988). Pessimistic explanatory style is a risk factor for physical illness: A thirty-five-year longitudinal study. *Journal of Personality and Social Psychology*, 55, 23–7.

Petty, R. and Cacioppo, J.T. (1986). *Communication and persuasion: Central and peripheral routes to attitude change*. New York: Springer.

Petty, R., Wells, G.L. and Brock, T.C. (1976). Distraction can enhance or reduce yielding to propaganda: Thought disruption versus effort justification. *Journal of Personality and Social Psychology*, 34, 874–84.

Petty, R., Cacioppo, J.T. and Goldman, R. (1981). Personal involvement as a determinant of argument-based persuasion. *Journal of Personality and Social Psychology*, 41, 847–55.

Polich, J.M., Armor, D.J. and Braiker, H.B. (1981). *The course of alcoholism*, New York: John Wiley.

Polivy, J. (1976). Perception of calories and regulation of intake in restrained and unrestrained subjects. *Addictive Behavior*, 1, 237–43.

Polivy, J. and Herman, C.P. (1976). Effects of alcohol on eating behavior: Influence of mood and perceived intoxication. *Journal of Abnormal Psychology*, 85, 601–606.

Polivy, J. and Herman, C.P. (1987). Diagnosis and treatment of normal eating. *Journal of Consulting and Clinical Psychology*, 28, 341–3.

Pomerleau, O.F. and Pomerleau, C.S. (1989). A biobehavioral perspective on smoking. In T. Ney and A. Gale (Eds), *Smoking and behavior*, pp. 69–90. Chichester: John Wiley.

Pomerleau, O.F., Pertschuk, M., Adkins, D. and Brady, J.P. (1978). A comparison of behavioral and traditional treatment for middle income problem drinkers. *Journal of Behavioral Medicine*, 1, 187–200.

Pooling Project Research Group (1978). *Relationship of blood pressure, serum cholesterol, smoking habit, relative weight and ECG-abnormality to incidence of major coronary events: Final report of the Pooling Project*. American Heart Association Monographs No. 60. Dallas, TX: American Heart Association.

Powell, K.E., Thompson, P.D., Caspersen, C.J. and Kendrick, J.S. (1987). Physical activity and the incidence of coronary heart disease. *Annual Review of Public Health*, 8, 253–87.

Puska, P., Nissinen, A., Tuomilehto, J., Salonen, J.T., Koskela, K., McAlister, A., Kottke, T.E., Maccoby, N. and Farquhar, J.W. (1985). The community-based strategy to prevent coronary heart disease: Conclusions from ten years of the North Karelia Project. In L. Breslow, J.E. Fielding and L.B. Lave (Eds), *Annual Review of Public Health*, Vol. 6, pp. 147–94. Palo Alto, CA: Annual Reviews Inc.

Rabkin, J.G. and Struening, E.L. (1976). Life events, stress, and illness. *Science*, 194, 1013–20.

Rahe, R.H. (1968). Life change measurement as a predictor of illness. *Proceedings of the Royal Society of Medicine*, 61, 124–6.

Rahe, R.H. and Lind, E. (1971). Psychosocial factors and sudden cardiac death: A pilot study. *Journal of Psychosomatic Research*, 15, 19–24.

Rahe, R.H. and Paasikivi, J. (1971). Psychosocial factors and myocardial infarction. II. An outpatient study in Sweden. *Journal of Psychosomatic Research*, 15, 33–9.

Rahe, R.H., Romo, M. and Bennett, L. (1974). Recent life changes, myocardial infarction and abrupt coronary death. Studies in Helsinki. *Archives of Internal Medicine*, 133, 222–8.

Raphael, B. (1986). *When disaster strikes*. London: Hutchinson.

Reich, W.P., Parrella, D.P. and Filstead, W.J. (1988). Unconfounding the hassles scale: External sources *vs* internal responses to stress. *Journal of Behavioral Medicine*, 11, 239–50.

Reinish, J.M., Sanders, S.A. and Ziemba-Davis, M. (1988). The study of sexual behavior in relation to the transmission of human immuno-deficiency virus: Caveats and recommendations. *American Psychologist*, 43, 921–7.

Remington, P.L., Forman, M.R., Gentry, E.M., Marks, J.S., Hogelin, G.C. and Trowbridge, F.L. (1985). Current smoking trends in the United States: The 1981–1983 Behavioral Risk Factor surveys. *Journal of the American Medical Association*, 253, 2975–8.

Rhodewalt, F. and Zone, J.B. (1989). Appraisal of life change, depression and illness in hardy and nonhardy women. *Journal of Personality and Social Psychology*, 56, 81–8.

Richard, R. and van der Pligt, J. (1991). Factors affecting condom use among adolescents. In *Journal of Community and Applied Social Psychology*, 1, 105–116.

Riddle, P.K. (1980). Attitudes, beliefs, behavioral intentions, and behaviors of men and women toward regular jogging. *Research Quarterly for Exercise and Sport*, 51, 663–74.

Riley, D.M., Sobell, L.D., Leo, G.I., Sobell, M. and Klajner, F. (1987). Behavioral treatment of alcohol: A review and a comparison of behavioral and nonbehavioral studies. In M. Wilcox (Ed.), *Treatment and prevention of alcohol problems: A resource manual*, pp. 73–115. San Diego, CA: Academic Press.

Rippetoe, P.A. and Rogers, R.W. (1987). Effects of components of protection–motivation theory on adaptive and maladaptive coping with a health threat. *Journal of Personality and Social Psychology*, 52, 596–604.

Robertson, K., Kelley, A., O'Neill, B., Wixom, C., Eisworth, R. and Hadon, W., Jr (1974). A controlled study of the effect of television messages on safety belt use. *American Journal of Public Health*, 64, 1071–80.

Robertson, L.S. (1978). The seat belt use law in Ontario: Effects on actual use. *Canadian Journal of Public Health*, 70, 599–603.

Robertson, L.S. (1984). Behavior and injury prevention: Whose behavior? In J.D. Matarazzo, S.M. Weis, J.A. Herd, N.E. Miller and S.M. Weiss (Eds), *Behavioral health*, pp. 980–9. New York: John Wiley.

Robertson, L.S. (1986). Behavioral and environmental interventions for reducing motor vehicle trauma. In L. Breslow, J.E. Fielding and L.B. Lave (Eds), *Annual review of public health*, pp. 13–34. Palo Alto, CA: Annual Reviews Inc.

Robertson, L.S. (1987). Injury prevention: Limits to self-protective behavior. In N.D. Weinstein (Ed.), *Taking care*, pp. 280–97. New York: Cambridge University Press.

Rodin, J. (1981). Current status of the internal–external hypothesis for obesity. *American Psychologist*, 36, 361–72.

Rodin, J., Slochower, J. and Fleming, B. (1977). The effects of degree of obesity, age of onset, and energy deficit on external responsiveness. *Journal of Comparative and Physiological Psychology*, 91, 586–97.

Rogers, R.W. (1983). Cognitive and physiological processes in fear appeals and attitude change: A revised theory of protection motivation. In J.T. Cacioppo and R.E. Petty (Eds), *Social psychophysiology: A source book*, pp. 153–76. New York: Guilford Press.

Rogers, R.W. (1985). Attitude change and information integration in fear appeals. *Psychological Reports*, 56, 179–82.

Rogers, R.W. and Mewborn, C.R. (1976). Fear appeals and attitude change: Effects of noxiousness, probability of occurrence, and the efficacy of coping responses. *Journal of Personality and Social Psychology*, 34, 54–61.

Rohde, P., Lewinsohn, P.M., Tilson, M. and Sealey, J.R. (1990). Dimensionality of coping and its relation to depression. *Journal of Personality and Social Psychology*, 58, 499–511.

Roizen, J. (1982). Estimating alcohol involvement in serious events. In National Institute of Alcohol Abuse and Alcoholism (Ed.), *Alcohol consumption and related problems*, pp. 179–219. Washington, DC: DHHS.

Rosenberg, H. (1993). Prediction of controlled drinking by alcoholics and problem drinkers. *Psychological Bulletin*, 113, 129–39.

Rosenberg, M.J. (1960). An analysis of affective–cognitive consistency. In C.I. Hovland and M.J. Rosenberg (Eds), *Attitude organization and change*, pp. 15–64. New Haven, CT: Yale University Press.

Rosenberg, M.J. and Hovland, C.I. (1960). Cognitive, affective, and behavioral components of attitudes. In I. Hovland and M.J. Rosenberg (Eds), *Attitude organization and change*, pp. 1–14. New Haven, CT: Yale University Press.

Rosenstock, I. (1974). The health belief model and preventive health behavior. *Health Education Monographs*, 2, 354–86.

Rosenthal, B.S. and Marx, R.D. (1978). Differences in eating patterns of successful and unsuccessful dieters, untreated overweight and normal weight individuals. *Addictive Behavior*, 3, 129–34.

Ross, C.E. and Mirowsky, J. (1979). A comparison of life-event weighting schemes: Change, undesirability, and effect-proportional indices. *Journal of Health and Social Behavior*, 20, 166–77.

Rothenberg, R.B. and Koplan, J.P. (1990). Chronic disease in the 1990s. *Annual Review of Public Health*, 11, 267–96.

Rotter, J.B., Seeman, M. and Liverant, S. (1962). Internal *vs* external locus of control of reinforcement: A major variable in behavior therapy. In N.F. Washburne (Ed.), *Decisions, values, and groups*, pp. 473–516. Oxford: Pergamon Press.

Ruberman, W., Weinblatt, E., Goldberg, J.D. and Chaudhary, B.S. (1984). Psychosocial influences on mortality after myocardial infarction. *New England Journal of Medicine*, 311, 552–9.

Ruderman, A.J. (1986). Dietary restraint: A theoretical and empirical review. *Psychological Bulletin*, 99, 247–62.

Ruderman, A.J. and Christensen, H.C. (1983). Restraints theory and its applicability to overweight individuals. *Journal of Abnormal Psychology*, 92, 210–15.

Russell, M.A.H., Wilson, C., Feyerabend, C. and Cole, P.V. (1976). Effect of nicotine chewing-gum on smoking behaviour and as an aid to cigarette withdrawal. *British Medical Journal*, 2, 391–3.

Russell, M.A.H., Wilson, C., Taylor, C. and Baker, C.D. (1979). Effect of general practitioners' advice against smoking. *British Medical Journal*, 2, 231–5.

Rzewnicki, R. and Forgays, D. (1987). Recidivism and self-cure of smoking and obesity: An attempt to replicate. *American Psychologist*, 42, 97–100.

Salber, E.J., Reed, R.B., Harrison, S.V. and Green, J.H. (1963). Smoking behavior, recreational activities and attitudes toward smoking among Newton secondary school children. *Pediatrics*, 32, 911–18.

Salonen, J.T., Puska, P. and Tuomilehto, J. (1982). Physical activity and risk of myocardial infarction, cerebral stroke and death: A longitudinal study in eastern Finland. *American Journal of Epidemiology*, 115, 526–37.

Sanders, C. (1993). Risk factors in bereavement outcome. In M. Stroebe, W. Stroebe and R. Hansson (Eds), *Handbook of bereavement*, pp. 255–67. New York: Cambridge University Press.

Sarafino, E.P. (1990). *Health psychology: Biopsychosocial interactions.* New York: John Wiley.

Sarason, B.R., Shearin, E.N., Pierce, G.R. and Sarason, I.G. (1987). Interrelationships among social support measures: Theoretical and practical implications. *Journal of Personality and Social Psychology*, 52, 813–32.

Sarason, B.R., Sarason, I.G. and Pierce, G.R. (1990). Traditional views of social support and their impact on assessment. In B.R. Sarason, I.G. Sarason and G.R. Pierce (Eds), *Social support: An interactional view*, pp. 9–25. New York: John Wiley.

Sarason, I.G., Johnson, J.H. and Siegel, J.M. (1978). Assessing the impact of life changes: Development of the Life Experience Survey. *Journal of Consulting and Clinical Psychology*, 46, 932–46.

Sarason, I.G., Levine, H.M., Basham, R.B. and Sarason, B.R. (1983). Assessing social support: The social support questionnaire. *Journal of Personality*, 44, 127–39.

Schaalma, H., Kok, G. and Peters, L. (1993). Determinants of consistent condom use by adolescents: The impact of experience of sexual intercourse. *Health Education Research*, 8, 255–69.

Schachter, S. (1959). *The psychology of affiliation*. Stanford, CA: Stanford University Press.

Schachter, S. (1977). Nicotine regulation in heavy and light smokers. *Journal of Experimental Psychology: General*, 106, 5–12.

Schachter, S. (1978). Pharmacological and psychological determinants of smoking. *Annals of Internal Medicine*, 88, 104–114.

Schachter, S. (1982). Recidivism and self-cure of smoking and obesity. *American Psychologist*, 37, 436–44.

Schachter, S. and Gross, L.P. (1968). Manipulated time and eating behavior. *Journal of Personality and Social Psychology*, 10, 98–106.

Schachter, S., Kozlowski, L.T. and Silverstein, B. (1977a). Effects of urinary pH on secret smoking. *Journal of Experimental Psychology: General*, 106, 13–19.

Schachter, S., Silverstein, B. and Perlick, D. (1977b). Psychological and pharmacological explanations of smoking under stress. *Journal of Experimental Psychology: General*, 106, 31–40.

Scheier, M.F. and Carver, C.S. (1985). Optimism, coping and health: Assessment and implications of generalized outcome expectancies. *Health Psychology*, 4, 219–47.

Scheier, M.F. and Carver, C.S. (1987). Dispositional optimism and physical well-being: The influence of generalized outcome expectancies on health. *Journal of Personality*, 55, 169–210.

Scheier, M.F., Weintraub, J.K. and Carver, C.S. (1986). Coping with stress: Divergent strategies of optimists and pessimists. *Journal of Personality and Social Psychology*, 51, 1257–64.

Scheier, M.F., Matthews, K.A., Owens, J., Magovern, G.J., Lefebvre, R.C., Abbott, R.A. and Carver, C.S. (1989). Dispositional optimism and recovery from coronary artery bypass surgery: The beneficial effects on physical and psychological well-being. *Journal of Personality and Social Psychology*, 57, 1024–40.

Schifter, D.E. and Ajzen, I. (1985). Intention, perceived control, and weight loss: An application of the theory of planned behavior. *Journal of Personality and Social Psychology*, 49, 843–851.

Schmidt, W. (1977). Cirrhosis and alcohol consumption: An epidemiological perspective. In G. Edwards and M. Grant (Eds), *Alcoholism: New knowledge and new responses*, pp. 15–47. London: Croom Helm.

Schmidt, W. and de Lint, J. (1970). Estimating the prevalence of alcoholism from alcohol consumption and mortality data. *Quarterly Journal of Studies on Alcohol*, 31, 957–64.

Schmied, L.A. and Lawler, K.A. (1986). Hardiness, Type A behavior, and the stress–illness relationship in working women. *Journal of Personality and Social Psychology*, 51, 1218–23.

Schoenbach, V.J., Kaplan, B.H., Fredman, L. and Kleinbaum, D.G. (1986). Social ties and mortality in Evans County, Georgia. *American Journal of Epidemiology*, 123, 577–91.

Schotte, D.E., Cools, J. and McNally, R.J. (1990). Film induced negative affect triggers overeating in restrained eaters. *Journal of Abnormal Psychology*, 99, 317–20.

Schroeder, D.H. and Costa, P.T., Jr (1984). Influence of life events' stress on physical illness: Substantive effects on methodological floors? *Journal of Personality and Social Psychology*, 46, 853–63.

Schwartz, J.L. (1987). *Smoking cessation methods: The United States and Canada, 1978–1985*. Division of Cancer Prevention and Control, National Cancer Institute, US Department of Health and Human Services, Public Health Service. NIH Publication No. 87–2940. Washington, DC: US Government Printing Office.

Schwarzer, R. and Leppin, A. (1989a). *Sozialer Rückhalt und Gesundheit: Eine Meta-Analyse*. Göttingen: Hogrefe.

Schwarzer, R. and Leppin, A. (1989b). Social support and health: A meta-analysis. *Psychology and Health: An International Journal*, 3, 1–15.

Segal, P., Rifkind, B.M. and Schull, W.J. (1982). Genetic factors in lipoprotein variation. *Epidemiology Reviews*, 4, 137–60.

Seibold, D.R. and Roper, R.E. (1979). Psychosocial determinants of health care intentions: Test of the Triandis and Fishbein models. In D. Nimmo (Ed.), *Communication yearbook 3*, pp. 625–43. New Brunswick, NJ: Transaction Books.

Seligman, M.E.P. (1975). *Helplessness*. San Francisco, CA: W.H. Freeman.

Selye, H. (1976). *The stress of life*, 2nd edn. New York: McGraw-Hill.

Shaper, A.G., Wannamethee, G. and Walker, M. (1988). Alcohol and morality in British men: Explaining the U-shaped curve. *Lancet*, 3, 1267–73.

Shiffman, S. (1982). Relapse following smoking cessation: A situational analysis. *Journal of Consulting and Clinical Psychology*, 50, 71–86.

Shiffman, S., Read, L., Maltese, J., Rapkin, D. and Jarvik, M.E. (1985). Preventing relapse in ex-smokers: a self-management approach. In G.A. Marlatt and J.R. Gordon (Eds), *Relapse prevention*, pp. 472–520. New York: Guilford.

Simopoulos, A.P. (1986). Obesity and body weight standards. In L. Breslow, J.E. Fielding and L.B. Lave (Eds), *Annual review of public health*, Vol. 7, pp. 475–92. Palo Alto, CA: Annual Reviews Inc.

Sims, E.A.H. and Horton, E.S. (1968). Endocrine and metabolic adaptation to obesity and starvation. *American Journal of Clinical Nutrition*, 21, 1455–70.

Sjöström, L. (1980). Fat cells and body weight. In A.J. Stunkard (Ed.), *Obesity*. Philadelphia, PA: W.B. Saunders.

Smetana, J.G. and Adler, N.E. (1980). Fishbein's value × expectancy model: An examination of some assumptions. *Personality and Social Psychology Bulletin*, 6, 89–96.

Smith, T.W., Pope, M.K., Rhodewalt, F. and Poulton, J.L. (1989). Optimism, neuroticism, coping, and symptom reports: An alternative interpretation of the Life Orientation Test. *Journal of Personality and Social Psychology*, 56, 640–48.

Society of Actuaries (1960). *Build and blood pressure study, 1959*. Chicago, IL: Society of Actuaries.

Society of Actuaries and Association of Life Insurance Medical Directors of America (1979). *Build study*. Chicago, IL: Society of Actuaries.

Sonstroem, R.J. (1978). Physical estimation and attraction scales: Rationale and research. *Medicine and Science in Sports*, 10, 97–102.

Sonstroem, R.J. (1988). Psychological models. In R.K. Dishman (Ed.), *Exercise adherence: Its impact on public health*, pp. 125–53. Champaign, IL: Human Kinetics.

Sonstroem, R.J. and Kampper, K.P. (1980). Prediction of athletic participation in middle school males. *Research Quarterly for Exercise and Sport*, 51, 685–94.

Spielberger, C.D. (1986). Psychological determinants of smoking behavior. In L.D. Tollison (Ed.), *Smoking and society*, pp. 89–132. Lexington, MA: Heath.

Spring, F.L., Sipich, J.F., Trimble, R.W. and Goeckner, D.J. (1978). Effects of contingency and non-contingency contracts in the context of a self-control-oriented smoking modification program. *Behavior Therapy*, 9, 967–8.

Stallones, R.A. (1983). Ischemic heart disease and lipids in blood and diet. *Annual Review of Nutrition*, 3, 155–85.

Stalonas, P.M., Johnson, W.G. and Christ, M. (1978). Behavior modification for obesity: The evaluation of exercise, contingency management and program adherence. *Journal of Consulting and Clinical Psychology*, 46, 463–9.

Stanton, A.L. and Snoder, P.R. (1993). Coping with a breast cancer diagnosis: A prospective study. *Health Psychology*, 12, 16–23.

Stein, M., Keller, S.E. and Schleifer, S.J. (1985). Stress and immunomodulation: The role of depression and neuroendocrine function. *Journal of Immunology*, 135, 827–33 (suppl.).

Steinberg, H. and Sykes, E.A. (1985). Introduction to symposium on endorphins and behavioral processes: Review of literature on endorphins and exercise. *Pharmacology, Biochemistry and Behavior*, 23, 857–62.

Stokes, J.P. (1983). Predicting satisfaction with social support from social network structure. *American Journal of Community Psychology*, 11, 141–52.

Strain, G.W., Strain, J.J., Zumoff, B. and Knittle, J. (1984). Do fat cells' morphometrics predict weight loss? *International Journal of Obesity*, 8, 53–9.

Striegel-Moore, R. and Rodin, J. (1986). The influence of psychological variables in obesity. In K.D. Brownell and J.P. Foreyt (Eds), *Handbook of eating disorders*, pp. 99–121. New York: Basic Books.

Stroebe, M. (1992). Coping with bereavement: A review of the grief work hypothesis. *Omega*, 26, 19–42.

Stroebe, M. and Stroebe, W. (1993). Mortality of bereavement: A review. In M. Stroebe, W. Stroebe and R. Hansson (Eds), *Handbook of bereavement*, pp. 175–95. New York: Cambridge University Press.

Stroebe, M., Stroebe, W. and Hansson, R. (Eds) (1993). *Handbook of bereavement*. New York: Cambridge University Press.

Stroebe, W. and Stroebe, M.S. (1987). *Bereavement and health*. New York: Cambridge University Press.

Stroebe, W. and Stroebe, M.S. (1993). Determinants of adjustment to bereavement in younger widows and widowers. In M.S. Stroebe, W. Stroebe and R. Hansson (Eds), *Handbook of bereavement*, pp. 208–226. New York: Cambridge University Press.

Stroebe, W., Stroebe, M.S. and Domittner, G. (1988). Individual and situational differences in recovery from bereavement: A risk group identified. *Journal of Social Issues*, 44, 143–58.

Stuart, R.B. and Davis, B. (1972). *Slim chance in a fat world*. Champaign, IL: Research Press.

Stulb, S.C., McDonough, J.R., Geenberg, B.G. and Hames, C.G. (1965). The relationship of nutrient intake and exercise to serum cholesterol level in white males in Evans County, Georgia. *American Journal of Clinical Nutrition*, 16, 238–42.

Stunkard, A.J. (1984). The current status of treatment for obesity in adults. In A.J. Stunkard and E. Stellar (Eds), *Eating and its disorders*, pp. 157–74. New York: Raven Press.

Stunkard, A.J. (1986). The control of obesity: Social and community perspectives. In K.D. Brownell and J.P. Foreyt (Eds), *Handbook of eating disorders*, pp. 213–28. New York: Basic Books.

Stunkard, A.J. and Koch, C. (1964). The interpretation of gastric motility: I. Apparent bias in the reports of hunger by obese persons. *Archives of Genetic Psychiatry*, 11, 74–82.

Stunkard, A.J., Levine, H. and Fox, S. (1970). The management of obesity: Patient self-help and medical treatment. *Archives of Internal Medicine*, 125, 1367–73.

Stunkard, A.J., Sorensen, T.I.A., Hanis, C., Teasdale, T.W., Chakraborty, R., Schull, W.J. and Schulsinger, F. (1986). An adoption study of human obesity. *New England Journal of Medicine*, 314, 193–8.

Sutton, S.R. (1982). Fear-arousing communications: A critical examination of theory and research. In J.R. Eiser (Ed.), *Social psychology and behavioral medicine*, pp. 303–337. Chichester: John Wiley.

Sutton, S.R. (1987). Social-psychological approaches to understanding addictive behaviours: Attitude–behaviour and decision-making models. *British Journal of Addiction*, 82, 355–70.

Sutton, S.R. and Hallett, R. (1989). Understanding the effect of fear-arousing communications: The role of cognitive factors and amount of fear aroused. *Journal of Behavioral Medicine*, 11, 353–60.

Sweeney, P., Anderson, K. and Bailey, S. (1986). Attributional style in depression: A meta-analytic review. *Journal of Personality and Social Psychology*, 50, 774–91.

Tajfel, H. (1978). Social categorization, social identity and social comparison, in H. Tajfel (Ed.) *Differentiation between Social Groups*. London: Academic Press.

Taylor, S.E. (1991). *Health psychology*, 2nd edn. New York: McGraw-Hill.

Terborg, J.R. (1988). The organisation as a context for health promotion. In S. Spacapn and S. Oskamp (Eds), *The social psychology of health*, pp. 129–74. Newbury Park, CA: Sage.

Terris, M. (1967). Epidemiology of cirrhosis of the liver: National mortality data. *American Journal of Public Health*, 57, 2076–88.

Theorell, T. and Rahe, R.H. (1971). Psychosocial factors and myocardial infarction. I. An inpatient study in Sweden. *Journal of Psychosomatic Research*, 15, 25–31.

Theorell, T., Lind, E. and Floderus, B. (1975). The relationship of disturbing life changes and emotions to the early development of myocardial infarction and other serious illnesses. *International Journal of Epidemiology*, 4, 281–93.

Thompson, E.L. (1978). Smoking education programs, 1960–1976. *American Journal of Public Health*, 68, 250–57.

Thompson, J.K., Jarvie, G.J., Lahey, B.B. and Cureton, K.J. (1982). Exercise and Obesity: Etiology, Physiology and Intervention. *Psychological Bulletin*, 91, 55–79.

Thompson, P.D., Jeffery, R.W., Wing, R.R. and Wood, P.D. (1979). Unexpected degrees in plasma high density lipoprotein cholesterol with weight loss. *American Journal of Clinical Nutrition*, 32, 2016–21.

Tomkins, S.S. (1966). Psychological model for smoking behavior. *American Journal of Public Health*, 56, 17–20 (suppl. 2).

Trichopoulos, D., Kalandidi, A. and Sparros, L. (1983). Lung cancer and passive smoking: Conclusion of a Greek study (Letter). *Lancet*, 2, 677–8.

Tuck, M.L., Sowers, J., Dornfield, L., Kledzik, G. and Maxwell, M. (1981). The effect of weight reduction on blood pressure, plasma renin activity, and plasma aldosterone levels in obese patients. *New England Journal of Medicine*, 304, 930–33.

Turpeinen, O. (1979). Effect of cholesterol-lowering diet on mortality from coronary heart disease and other causes. *Circulation*, 59, 1–7.

Udry, J., Clark, L., Chase, C. and Levy, M. (1972). Can mass media advertising increase contraceptive use? *Family Planning Perspectives*, 4, 37–44.

US Department of Health and Human Services (1982). *The health consequences of smoking. Cancer: A report of the Surgeon-General.* Rockville, MD: Office on Smoking and Health.

US Department of Health and Human Services (1985). *Fact book fiscal year 1985.* Bethesda, MD: National Heart, Lung and Blood Institute.

US Department of Health and Human Services (1986). *The health consequences of involuntary smoking: A report of the Surgeon-General.* Office on Smoking and Health. DHHS Publication No. (CDC) 87–8398. Washington, DC: US Government Printing Office.

US Surgeon-General (1984). *The health consequences of smoking: Chronic obstructive lung disease.* Washington, DC: US Government Printing Office.

Vaillant, G.E. (1983). *The natural history of alcoholism.* Cambridge, MA: Harvard University Press.

Valois, P., Desharnais, R. and Godin, G. (1988). A comparison of the Fishbein and the Triandis attitudinal models for the prediction of exercise intention and behavior. *Journal of Behavioral Medicine,* 11, 459–72.

van den Putte, B. (1991). 20 years of the theory of reasoned action of Fishbein and Ajzen: A meta-analysis. Unpublished manuscript. University of Amsterdam.

van Griensven, G.J.P., de Vroome, E.M.M., Tielman, R.A.P., Goudsmit, J., de Wolf, F. and Coutinho, R.A. (1988). Veranderingen in anogenitaal seksueel contact en condoomgebruik afhankelijk van relatiepatroon en HIV-ab serodiagnose. *Tijdschrift voor Sociale Gezondheidszoig,* 66, 157–60.

Van Itallie, T.B. (1979). Obesity: Adverse effects on health and longevity. *American Journal of Clinical Nutrition,* 32, 2723–33.

Vinokur, A. and Selzer, M. (1975). Desirable *vs* undesirable life events: The relationship to stress and mental distress. *Journal of Personality and Social Psychology,* 32, 329–37.

Vinokur-Kaplan, D. (1978). To have – or not to have – another child: Family planning attitudes, intentions, and behavior. *Journal of Applied Social Psychology,* 18, 710–30.

Volkmar, F.R., Stunkard, A.J., Woolston, J. and Bailey, B.A. (1981). High attrition rates in commercial weight reduction programs. *Archives of Internal Medicine,* 141, 426–8.

Wadden, T.A. and Bell, S.T. (1990). Obesity. In A.S. Bellack, M. Hersen and A.E. Kazdin (Eds), *International handbook of behavior modification and therapy,* 2nd edn, pp. 449–73. New York: Plenum Press.

Wadden, T.A. and Stunkard, A.J. (1986). A controlled trial of very-low-calorie diet in the treatment of obesity. *Journal of Consulting and Clinical Psychology,* 54, 482–8.

Wadden, T.A., Stunkard, A.J. and Brownell, K.D. (1983). Very low caloric diets: Their efficacy, safety and future. *Annals of Internal Medicine*, 99, 675–84.

Waller, J.A. (1987). Injury: Conceptual shifts and preventive implications. *Annual Review of Public Health*, 8, 21–49.

Wallston, B.S. and Wallston, K.A. (1981). Social psychological models of health and behavior: An examination and integration. In G. Sanders and J. Suls (Eds), *The social psychology of health and illness*, pp. 65–95. Hillsdale, NJ: Laurence Erlbaum Associates Inc.

Walsh, D.C. and Gordon, N.P. (1986). Legal approaches to smoking deterrence. In L. Breslow, J.E. Fielding and L.B. Lave (Eds), *Annual review of public health*, Vol. 7, pp. 127–49. Palo Alto, CA: Annual Reviews Inc.

Warner, K.E. (1981). Cigarette smoking in the 1970's: The impact of the anti-smoking campaigns on consumption. *Science*, 211, 729–31.

Warner, K.E. (1986). Smoking and health implications of a change in the federal cigarette excise tax. *Journal of the American Medical Association*, 255, 1028–32.

Watson, D. and Pennebaker, J.W. (1989). Health complaints, stress, and distress: Exploring the central role of negative effectivity. *Psychological Review*, 96, 234–54.

Watson, J.B. and Raynor, R. (1920). Conditioned emotional reactions. *Journal of Experimental Psychology*, 3, 1–14.

Weinberger, M., Hiner, S.L. and Tierney, W.M. (1987). In support of hassles as measures of stress in predicting health outcomes. *Journal of Behavioral Medicine*, 10, 19–31.

Weinstein, M.C. and Stason, W.B. (1985). Cost-effectiveness of interventions to prevent or treat coronary heart disease. In L. Breslow, J.E. Fielding and L.B. Lave (Eds), *Annual reviews of public health*, Vol. 6, pp. 41–64. Palo Alto, CA: Annual Reviews Inc.

Weinstein, N.D. (1987). Unrealistic optimism about susceptibility to health problems: Conclusions from a community-wide sample. *Journal of Behavioral Medicine*, 10, 481–500.

Wiens, A.N. and Menustik, C.E. (1983). Treatment outcome and patient characteristics in an aversion therapy program for alcoholism. *American Psychologist*, 38, 1089–96.

Wilbur, C.S., Hartwell, T.D. and Piserchia, P.V. (1986). The Johnson & Johnson LIVE FOR LIFE Program: Its organization and evaluation plan. In M.F. Cataldo and T.J. Coates (Eds), *Health and industry: A behavioral medicine perspective*, pp. 338–50. New York: John Wiley.

Wilson, G.T. (1978). Methodological considerations in treatment outcome research on obesity. *Journal of Consulting and Clinical Psychology*, 46, 687–702.

Wilson, M. and Baker, S. (1987). Structural approach to injury control. *Journal of Social Issues*, 43, 73–86.

Winkelstein, W., Samuel, M., Padian, N., Wiley, J., Lang, W., Anderson, R. and Levy, J. (1987). The San Francisco men's health study: III. Reduction in HIV transmission among gay and bisexual men, 1982–86. *American Journal of Public Health*, 76, 685–9.

Wood, W. and Kallgren, C.A. (1988). Communicator attributes and persuasion: Recipients' access to attitude-relevant information in memory. *Personality and Social Psychology Bulletin*, 14, 172–82.

Wooley, S.C., Wooley, O.W. and Dyrenforth, S.R. (1979). Theoretical, practical and social issues in behavioral treatments of obesity. *Journal of Applied Behavior Analysis*, 12, 3–25.

World Health Organization (1982). *Prevention of coronary heart disease: A report of a WHO expert committee*, p. 53. Geneva: World Health Organization.

Zarski, J.J. (1984). Hassles and health: A replication. *Health Psychology*, 3, 243–51.

AUTHOR INDEX

SUBJECT INDEX